Contents

Preface

Nothing is rich but the inexhaustible wealth of
nature. She shows us only surfaces, but she is a
million fathoms deep.

Ralph Waldo Emerson

THE DATABANK

To the neophyte, surgery is the excitement of the operating room. This
elation soon yields to the reality of the vast, always changing, body of
knowledge required to care for the surgical patient. Maintaining this mental
databank is no easy task; we hope this book will help.

You will quickly discover that this book is not meant to be read through
from cover to cover. Instead, for each chapter, scan the material to assess the
surface, then mentally try to expand the "bare facts" outline into understand-
able prose to explore the depths. This method should help fix the information
in your mind. It will also expose areas which you do not fully comprehend.
For these areas, consult the selected bibliograhpy.

**The medical student should concentrate on pathophysiology, diagnosis
and indications for surgical intervention, while the resident must also
understand details of operative procedures and potential complications.**

A set of well-tested multiple choice questions follows each section
to allow reinforcement of the newly-acquired knowledge by its immediate use in deductive reasoning concerning patient management. It
is most effective to consult each chapter upon encountering a patient
with that condition.

EXPANDING THE DATABANK

Current information for expansion of the databank should be selected from at
least two of the following major surgical journals* read monthly:

*Prices given for journals and books are for students and residents in the United States in
1983.

American Journal of Surgery ($26)
    875 Third Avenue, New York, New York 10022

Annals of Surgery ($28)
    Journal Fulfillment Department; Lippincott/Harper, 2350 Virginia
    Avenue, Hagerstown, Maryland 21740

Archives of Surgery ($24 or included in AMA membership)
    535 North Dearborn Street, Chicago, Illinois 60610

British Journal of Surgery ($130)
    John Wright PSG Inc., 545 Great Road, P.O. Box 6, Littleton,
    Massachusetts 01460

Surgery ($31.60)
    C.V. Mosby Co., Circulation Department, 11830 Westline Industrial
    Drive, St. Louis, Missouri 63141

Surgery, Gynecology & Obstetrics ($20)
    54 East Erie Street, Chicago, Illinois 60611

Any of the following will provide excellent commentary and organization emphasizing current controversies:

Selected Readings in General Surgery ($125 for over 2,400 pages yearly)
    McClelland RN (ed), University of Texas Southwestern Medical
    School, 5323 Harry Hines Boulevard, Dallas, Texas 75235
    A well chosen set of current and classical reprints together with
    excellent in-depth critique and review questions. Arranged by subject
    and mailed monthly.

Audio-Digest in Surgery ($119 for 24 tapes yearly)
    Audio-Digest Foundation, 1577 East Chevy Chase Drive,
    Glendale, California 91206
    Cassette tapes of current information in surgery by highly respected
    consultants. A good way to keep up with current information,
    especially while driving to the hospital.

Current Problems in Surgery ($39 for 12 issues yearly)
    Year Book Medical Publishers, 35 East Wacker Drive, Chicago,
    Illinois 60601
    Well organized and superbly written. Includes oral-type examination
    questions.

Surgical Clinical of North America ($36 for 6 issues yearly)
    W.B. Saunders Co., West Washington Square, Philadelphia,
    Pennsylvania 19105
    Excellent in-depth review articles in selected areas including an
    exhaustive bibliography.

If you have access to an Apple™ computer, clinical simulations based on the theoretical principles presented in this book are available:

HIPPOCRATES (floppy disks) ($150 for each set of 10 surgical
  simulations)
    Appleton-Century-Crofts, Department NM, 25 Van Zant Street,
    East Norwalk, Connecticut 06855

USING THE DATABANK (THE BOARDS)

The ultimate criterion of a surgeon's knowledge is his ability to manage the patient. A formal examination can measure this only indirectly, and is based on the assumption that a thorough understanding of theory is a prerequisite for good patient care. Hopefully, the outline provided here will help both the student (in the NMB, FLEX, or ECFMG) and the surgical resident (in the in-training, qualifying and certifying examinations of the American Board of Surgery).

The following information is provided for the resident concerning board certification in General Surgery: (1) At the start of your residency, complete an application for the American College of Surgeons Candidate Group which can be obtained from The American College of Surgeons, 55 East Erie Street, Chicago, IL 60611; (2) Six months prior to completion of your approved Chief Residency, complete the preliminary evaluation form obtainable from The American Board of Surgery, 1617 John F. Kennedy Boulevard, Philadelphia, PA 19103; (3) The formal application for the boards will then be sent to you before June 1 of the year in which you wish to take the examination. Part I is a written multiple-choice test, including erasure-type patient management problems, given in late November or early December. Part II is the oral portion in which you will be examined by three groups of two examiners each for 30 minutes each. It is given about 6 times yearly and includes a projected slide examination for gross and microscopic surgical pathology.

ACKNOWLEDGMENTS

We wish to thank **students and residents** throughout the United States and Canada for their enthusiastic acceptance of the First Edition of this book. It is their pleas for expansion of the *databank* to include the remainder of *general surgery* that most encouraged us to prepare this second edition. We continue to welcome your comments and criticism.

The expert editorial guidance of Douglas Gall and Robert E. McGrath of Appleton-Century-Crofts was vital in permitting doubling of content while (hopefully) maintaining relevance and clarity with only a modest increase in size.

1. Thyroid

ANATOMY

1. Pseudolobulation: fibrous capsule with septae; false capsule: deep cervical fascia (See Fig. 1-1)
2. Pyramidal lobe: upward projection from isthmus, vestige of thyroglossal duct
3. Blood supply
   a. Superior thyroid arteries (from external carotid)
   b. Inferior thyroid arteries (from thyrocervical trunk of subclavian artery)
   c. Thyroidea ima (from aortic arch)
4. Venous drainage
   a. Superior and middle thyroid veins (from internal jugular)
   b. Inferior thyroid vein (from innominate)
5. Innervation
   a. Sympathetic (from cervical ganglion)
   b. Parasympathetic (from vagus via laryngeal nerves)
      i. Recurrent laryngeal nerve (motor to larynx): if injured → abductor laryngeal paralysis → cord will be in median position
      ii. Superior laryngeal nerve
         1) Internal branch (sensory) → injury → dysphagia and aspiration
         2) External branch (to cricothyroid muscle) → injury → early voice fatigue

PHYSIOLOGY

Iodine Metabolism
1. *Iodine* concentrated within gland, requires 0.1 mg/day to replace urinary losses (stimulated by TSH)
2. Form 3-monoiodotyrosine (MIT) and 3,5-diiodotyrosine (DIT)
3. Coupled to form T3 and T4, which are held in peptide linkage to thyroglobulin as intrafollicular colloid. Follicles (acini) lined with cuboidal epithelium, which become columnar when stimulated by TSH
4. Hydrolyzed by proteases and peptidases to T3 and T4 (enhanced by TSH)
5. T3 and T4 in plasma attach to plasma proteins (TBG and TBPA). T4:T3 = 10 to 20:1 because T3 is
   a. Less firmly protein bound
   b. More active
   c. Shorter lived

1

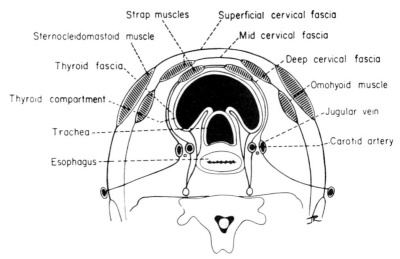

Figure 1-1 Anatomic relationships in cross section of the neck at the level of the thyroid gland. *(From Artz CP and Hardy JD (eds):* Management of Surgical Complications, *3rd Edt. W.B. Saunders Co., 1975, p 292, with permission.)*

6. T3 and T4 are conjugated in liver with glucuronic acid and excreted in bile. Some reabsorbed in bowel

Metabolic Effects of Thyroid Hormone
1. Increases oxygen consumption
2. Increases calorigenesis
3. Increases protein synthesis
4. Potentiates insulin effects on glycogen synthesis and glucose utilization
5. Decreases serum cholesterol and phospholipids

Hormonal Regulation

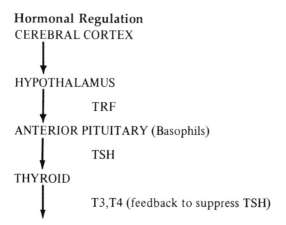

CEREBRAL CORTEX

↓

HYPOTHALAMUS

↓   TRF

ANTERIOR PITUITARY (Basophils)

↓   TSH

THYROID

↓   T3,T4 (feedback to suppress TSH)

DIAGNOSIS

1. Clinical findings
   a. Hyperthyroidism:
      i. Calorigenesis: heat intolerance, sweating, thirst, weight loss, increased appetite
      ii. Cardiovascular: tachycardia, atrial fibrillation, congestive heart failure, poor response to digoxin
      iii. Neuromuscular: excitable, hyperkinetic, emotionally unstable, insomnia, psychosis, muscle wasting due to myopathy
      iv. Skin: warm, moist, facial flushing, perspiration, fine hair, pretibial myxedema (associated with eye signs), gynecomastia (hepatic dysfunction)
      v. Gastrointestinal: diarrhea
      vi. Other: renal stones, demineralization of bone
   b. Hypothyroidism
   c. History of exposure to radiation
   d. Pressure symptoms (stridor)
   e. Mass moving with deglutition
   f. Mass in suprasternal notch
   g. Auscultation for bruits (hyperactive)
   h. Lymph nodes (Delphian node above thyroid associated with carcinoma or thyroiditis)
2. X-ray
   a. Miliary calcification → papillary carcinoma
   b. Extensive calcification → nodular goiter
   c. Compression of trachea
3. EKG (for thyrotoxicosis—atrial fibrillation)
4. Function tests
   a. Indirect
      i. BMR—oxygen uptake/body surface area
      ii. Cholesterol—hypothyroidism if over 300 mg percent
   b. Direct
      i. PBI (normal 3.5 to 8.0 μg percent)
      ii. I-131 uptake (normal 20 to 55 percent in 24 hours)
      iii. Estimation of plasma T3, T4, TSH
5. Thyroid scan (using I-131)
6. Thyroid antibody titers for Hashimoto's thyroiditis (not specific)
7. Needle or high-speed drill biopsy of mass (controversial): use 22 gauge needle for aspiration biopsy; larger needle may allow seeding of tumor in tract

THERAPY

Solitary Nodule, Nontoxic
1. Unilateral lobectomy and isthmusectomy
2. Malignancy in about one-third, increasing with decreasing age

3. Overall distribution
    a. Benign cold nodule—50 percent
    b. Malignant—29 percent
    c. Follicular adenoma—15 percent
    d. Hashimoto's thyroiditis—6 percent
    e. Congenital cyst, hematoma, Hodgkin's—3 percent
4. Cold vs. hot nodule on scan not diagnostic
5. Frozen section diagnosis: Some malignancies missed, which may require
   reoperation for total thyroidectomy
6. Postoperative thyroxin therapy may suppress recurrence of some lesions

Multinodular Goiter
1. Medical therapy
    a. Antithyroid drugs if toxic
        i. PTU, methimazole (interfere with synthesis of T3 and T4 by preventing
           oxidation of iodine to iodide)
        ii. RAI (dangerous because of possibility of subsequent carinoma or
            leukemia, hypothyroidism)
▶2. Indications for surgery: (Five M's)
    a. Malignancy: dominant or cold nodule; metastases proved to be thyroidal
       in origin; palpable nodes
    b. Mechanical: trachael compression
    c. Metabolic: non-response to hormone therapy
    d. Marred beauty: unslightly lump
    e. Mediastinal site
3. Procedure
    a. Subtotal thyroidectomy, or
    b. Total thyroidectomy (?)

▶COMPLICATIONS OF THRYOIDECTOMY ("THYROIDS")

1. Tetany: due to hypoparathyroidism; give calcium, Vitamin D
2. Hemorrhage: may require tracheostomy
3. Yell:
    a. Recurrent laryngeal nerve injury → cord fixed in midline → hoarseness,
       stridor (prevent by exposure during dissection)
    b. External branch of superior laryngeal nerve injury → early voice fatigue
4. Recurrent hyperthyroidism
5. Oesophageal damage
6. Infection
7. Death — 0.1 percent
8. Storm: thyroid storm (fever, tachycardia, tachypnea)

CANCER

Etiology
1. Irradiation in childhood (especially to thymus, 20-year latent period)

2. Familial (medullary carcinoma associated with increased calcitonin, pheochromocytoma, and mucosal neuromas)
3. Endemic goiter (due to increased TSH, debated)

Pathology
1. From follicular cells may be follicular, papillary, or anaplastic
2. From parafollicular cells are medullary
3. Lymphoma, rare

Characteristics

Papillary	Follicular	Medullary	Anaplastic
Youngest --Oldest			
Best prognosis --Worst prognosis			

Therapy
1. Total thyroidectomy (except lymphomas)
2. Lymphomas—chemo and radiotherapy
3. Inoperable tumors—radiation
4. Papillary and follicular
   a. Local nodes resection if frozen section positive
   b. I-131 200 mCi if postoperative scan positive
5. Anaplastic—postoperative irradiation to neck and upper mediastinum
6. Medullary—node dissection; irradiation for residual tumor

THYROIDITIS

1. Hashimoto's (most common)
   a. Autoimmune
   b. Associated with papillary carcinoma
   c. Painful enlargement, coughing
   d. Therapy is thyroid hormone
   e. Surgery only if nodule present
2. DeQuervain's disease
   a. Acute nonsuppurative thyroiditis
   b. Associated with upper respiratory infection
   c. Therapy is ASA, steroids
   d. Sometimes local radiation therapy
3. Riedel's struma
   a. Compression of trachea, esophagus, or recurrent laryngeal nerve
   b. Therapy is thyroid hormone suppression
   c. Surgery for compressive symptoms
4. Acute suppurative thyroiditis (least common): therapy is drainage of abscess

SELECTED BIBLIOGRAPHY

Britton KE, et al.: A strategy for thyroid function tests. Br Med J 3:350, 1975
De Groot LJ, Stanbury JB: The Thyroid and Its Diseases, 4th Edt. New York, Wiley, 1975
Foster RS: Morbidity and mortality after thyroidectomy. SGO 146:423, 1978
Sedgwick CI: Surgery of the Thyroid Gland. Philadelphia, Saunders, 1974

QUESTIONS

1. A 40-year-old clinically euthyroid female who as a child received irradiation for a condition involving her thymus now has an asymptomatic solitary nodule in the right lobe of her thyroid. I-131 scanning shows no uptake into this lesion. On sonogram it is a solid mass. Appropriate management at this time is:
   A. Total thyroidectomy
   B. Subtotal thyroidectomy
   C. Thyroid lobectomy
   D. Attempted needle aspiration
   E. Treatment with propylthiouracil

2. Which of the following types of thyroid pathology is most likely to be malignant?
   A. Cold nodule
   B. Follicular adenoma
   C. Hashimoto's thyroiditis
   D. DeQuervain's disease
   E. Riedel's struma

3. Voice fatigue occurring after thyroidectomy is most likely due to injury to which of the following nerves which may occur during a high ligation of the superior pole?
   A. External branch of the superior laryngeal nerve
   B. Internal branch of the superior laryngeal nerve
   C. Recurrent laryngeal nerve
   D. "Nonrecurrent" laryngeal nerve
   E. Hypoglossal nerve

4. Three hours after an otherwise uneventful thyroidectomy, a 50-year-old female develops a temperature of 105°F and her pulse rises to 140. Each of the following are components of appropriate therapy *except*:
   A. Epinephrine
   B. Propranolol
   C. Phenoxybenzamine
   D. Phenobarbital
   E. Steroids

5. Postoperative myxedema after thyroidectomy results in increased:
   A. Thyroid-stimulating hormone
   B. Serum thyroxine
   C. Serum triodothyronine

D. Basal metabolic rate
E. None of these

6. An 18-year-old female presents with a 1.5-cm nodule in the right supraclavicar area. It is removed and found to be well-differentiated normal thyroid tissue within a lymph node. This is most likely:
   A. Lateral aberrant thyroid
   B. Anaplastic cancer
   C. Hashimoto's thyroiditis
   D. Metastatic thyroid cancer
   E. A normal finding

7. In thyroid malignancies, psamomma bodies are characteristic of:
   A. Papillary carcinoma
   B. Medullary carcinoma
   C. Follicular carcinoma
   D. Hurthle cell adenocarcinoma
   E. Anaplastic carcinoma

8. The most frequent cause of hypothroidism is:
   A. Carcinoma
   B. Hashimoto's thyroiditis
   C. Riedel's struma
   D. Iatrogenic
   E. Nodular goiter

ANSWERS

1. **C** Solid solitary thyroid nodules will be malignant in 30 percent of cases and require lobectomy for diagnosis. Further therapy depends on the type of malignancy and the degree of involvement of lymph nodes. "Hot" nodules may be treated initially with suppression using thyroid hormones, but even with "hot" nodules, if they do not suppress, lobectomy is required because cancer is still a possibility. The previous history of exposure to irradiation is even more suggestive of malignancy.

2. **A** Cold nodules (that is, nodules not taking up radioactive iodine on thyroid scan) are quite likely to be malignant and require excision.

3. **A** The external branch of the superior laryngeal nerve is usually found in intimate proximity to the superior thyroid vessels. Consequences of injury to this nerve include losses of timbre and focus with heavy use of the voice. In contrast, injury to the recurrent laryngeal nerve, which is adjacent to the posteromedial aspect of the thyroid near the tracheoesophageal groove, results in immediate and permanent hoarseness. Whether injury to this nerve is best avoided by exposing or avoiding this nerve is an issue that is not completely settled.

4. **A** Very high fever and tachycardia following thyroidectomy suggests thyroid storm. Appropriate therapy includes propranolol (Inderal), a beta-blocker to inhibit the cardiovascular effects of the sudden thyroid release, iodine to inhibit further release of the hormone, oxygen, and

occasionally pheoxybenzamine, phenobarbital, or steroids. Epinephrine is contraindicated.

5. **A** The lack of feedback inhibition will result in a rise in TSH after thyroidectomy.

6. **D** In some cases, the primary thyroid cancer is too small to be noticed on physical examination. It is possible that lymph node metastases from well-differentiated papillary and follicular tumors may be the only clinical manifestations. They are histologically so similar to normal thyroid tissue that such metastatics were previously called "lateral aberrant thyroid." It is now known that these represent metastatic disease.

7. **A** Psamomma bodies are concentric layers of calcium deposits occurring with papillary cancer of the thyroid.

8. **D** Twenty-five percent of cases result from subtotal thyroidectomy, usually for Grave's disease. An additional large number result from radiotherapy for hyperthyroidism.

2. Parathyroid

ANATOMY

Size
1. Less than 30 mg each
2. Less than 5 mm widest diameter

Origin
1. Lower (travels)—3rd branchial pouch
2. Upper (stationary)—4th branchial pouch
3. May be located within thyroid lobe

Histology
1. Chief cells—produce parathyroid hormone (PTH)
2. Oxyphilic cells
3. "C" cells: from ultimobranchial bodies, produce calcitonin, also in thyroid and thymus

PHYSIOLOGY OF PTH:

Polypeptide that ↑ calcium and ↓ phosphate
1. Bone: dissolution of organic and inorganic components, inhibition of new bone formation
2. Kidney: increase of calcium reabsorption, inhibition of phosphate reabsorption
3. Intestinal mucosa: permits vitamin D-mediated calcium transport into duodenal and upper jejunal cells

HYPERPARATHYROIDISM—ETIOLOGY

Primary
1. Single adenoma or diffuse hyperplasia
2. Rarely carcinoma (1 percent)

Secondary
1. Chronic renal failure } Low calcium causes
2. Rickets, osteomalacia } chief cell hyperplasia

Tertiary
Late secondary when hyperplasia becomes autonomus

Pseudo
PTH produced by tumor such as squamous cell carcinoma of the lung or renal cell carcinoma

▶ **CLINICAL FINDINGS ("Stones, Bones, Abdominal Groans")**

1. Renal: colic, infections, stones, hematuria, azotemia
2. Bone: osteoporosis, osteitis fibrosa cystica, subperiosteal resorption
3. GI: nausea, anorexia, constipation
4. Neuromuscular: weakness, fatigue, mental changes

DIAGNOSIS

1. Consistently elevated serum calcium
2. Decreased tubular reabsorption of phosphate (TRP) after oral phosphate loading
3. Exclusion of
   a. Exogenous hypercalcemia (thiazides, milk-alkali, vitamin D)
   b. Non-PTH-mediated hypercalcemia (osseous malignancy, breast cancer, multiple myeloma, sarcoidosis, thyroid disease, immobilization)
4. Venous catheterization and radioimmunoassay for PTH (usually used only in complicated or previously operated cases)

ASSOCIATED CONDITIONS

1. Pancreatitis, peptic ulcer disease, hypertension
2. Multiple endocrine adenomatoses
   a. MEA_1 (Wermer's) = parathyroid, pituitary, pancreatic tumors
   b. MEA_2 (Sipple's) = parathyroid, medullary thyroid, medullary adrenal tumors

MEDICAL THERAPY

1. Inorganic phosphate; if surgery contraindicated
2. In acute hypercalcemic state
   a. Induce sodium diuresis with normal saline and furosemide
   b. Mithramycin

   c. Dialysis
   d. Semielective parathyroidectomy

SURGICAL THERAPY

Indications
1. All symptomatic cases, or if
2. Calcium consistently over 11 mg percent, or
3. Urinary calcium over 250 mg daily despite low calcium diet

Procedure
Careful search for all four glands, which *may* require
1. Division of superior thyroid vessels
2. Thyroid lobectomy
3. Dissection of tracheoesophageal grooves
4. Resection of carotid sheath
5. Superior mediastinal exploration 1 month later if hypercalcemia persists

Extent of Procedure
1. One gland enlarged—excise that gland
2. Two or more enlarged—subtotal parathyroidectomy (3½ glands removed). May autotransplant one gland into forearm or freeze in liquid nitrogen
3. Carcinoma—wide en-bloc resection, possible radical neck dissection (5-year survival is 50 percent)

Anatomical Landmark
Junction of inferior thyroid artery and recurrent laryngeal nerve; most inferior parathyroid glands lie below this junction and most superior parathyroids lie above it

Reexploration
1. Preoperative arteriogram and venous PTH studies
2. Reconfirm diagnosis
3. Stain intraoperatively with intravenous methylene blue

SELECTED BIBLIOGRAPHY

Burnett HF, et al.: Parathyroid autotransplantation. Arch Surg 112:373, 1977

Goldman L, et al.: The parathyroids: Progress, problems and practice. Curr Probl Surg, 8(8), 1971

Harrison TS, Thompson NW: Multiple endocrine adenomatoses: I and II. Curr Probl Surg 12(8), 1975

Wang CA: The anatomical basis of parathyroid surgery. Ann Surg 183:271, 1976

QUESTIONS

DIRECTIONS: For each of the questions or incomplete statements below, *one* or *more* of the answers or completions given is correct. Select:

    A   if only *1, 2, and 3* are correct
    B   if only *1 and 3* are correct
    C   if only *2 and 4* are correct
    D   if only *4* is correct
    E   if all are correct

A 42-year-old female with right flank pain and hematuria noted also unusual irritability, confusion, muscular aches, and anorexia. On physical examination, thick, dry fingernails and muscular hypotonicity were found. X-ray studies showed generalized bony demineralization and a calcified right renal stone. Serum calcium was 12.8 mg percent, phosphate 1.5 mg percent, and alkaline phosphatase moderately elevated.

1. If these biochemical abnormalities are due to primary hyperparathyroidism they result from:
   1. "Renal phosphate leak"
   2. Increased intestinal calcium reabsorption
   3. Increased renal tubular calcium reabsorption
   4. Bone dissolution
2. If this patient suddenly developed vomiting and bizarre mentation with a serum-calcium of 17 mg percent, accepted *immediate* therapy includes:
   1. Normal saline
   2. Thiazide diuretics
   3. Mithramycin
   4. Parathyroidectomy
3. Pseudohyperparathyroidism is associated with:
   1. Sarcoidosis
   2. Multiple myeloma
   3. Breast cancer
   4. Renal cell tumor
4. The MEA$_1$ syndrome should be considered if these findings are associated with:
   1. Bitemporal hemianopsia
   2. Elevated serum gastrin level
   3. Diabetes mellitus
   4. Pheochromocytoma
5. Findings associated with primary hyperparathyroidism are:
   1. Elevated serum amylase
   2. Peptic ulcer disease aggravated by antacids
   3. Hypertension relieved by parathyroidectomy
   4. Primary myopathy

6. Should neck exploration reveal both left parathyroids and only one right gland, which of the following should be considered:
   1. Resection of carotid sheath
   2. Right thyroid lobectomy
   3. Intravenous methylene blue
   4. Immediate median sternotomy
7. Indications for parathyroidectomy in secondary hyperparathyroidism due to chronic renal failure include:
   1. Pathologic fractures
   2. Progressive symptomatic hypercalcemia in patients with well-functioning renal allografts
   3. Intractable itching
   4. Symptomatic hypercalcemia despite medical therapy in patients on chronic maintenance hemodialysis
8. Indications for surgery in asymptomatic hyperparathyroidism include:
   1. Serum phosphate below 3 mg percent
   2. Urinary calcium over 250 mg daily despite low calcium diet
   3. Normocalcemia
   4. Serum calcium consistently over 11 mg percent

DIRECTIONS: Each of the questions or incomplete statements below is followed by five suggested answers or completions. Select the *one* that is *best* in each case.

---

9. Assume that primary hyperparathyroidism is well documented. Neck exploration reveals two enlarged parathyroids that appear to be chief-cell adenomas on frozen section. Further exploration reveals two normal-appearing glands. The procedure of choice is:
   A. Remove only the two abnormal glands
   B. Perform a total thyroidectomy
   C. Perform a subtotal parathyroidectomy
   D. Perform a mediastinal exploration
   E. None of these
10. In this case assume that a single parathyroid adenoma was found inferiorly in the left prevertebral space and removed. Postoperatively, hypercalcemia persists. A right thyroid arteriogram shows a blush lying inferior and posterior to the inferior border of the thyroid. Selective venous PTH studies are normal in all but two samples, thyroid ima vein and middle left innominate vein, which are significantly elevated. The most likely finding at reexploration is:
    A. Thyroid adenoma with normal parathyroids
    B. Hyperplasia of the three remaining parathyroids
    C. Hyperplasia of two parathyroids, one left and one right
    D. Left superior parathyroid adenoma
    E. Right superior parathyroid adenoma

ANSWERS

1. **E** All effects of PTH.
2. **B** Induce natrieuresis. Thiazides contraindicated. Parathyroidectomy is semielective.
3. **D** Others cause non-parathormone-mediated hypercalcemia.
4. **A** Pituitary lesions cause compression of optic chiasm. Pancreatic tumors may be beta or nonbeta. Pheochromocytoma is associated with MEA_2.
5. **A** Myopathy is secondary to electrolyte abnormalities. Amylase is elevated in pancreatitis.
6. **A** Sternotomy should be delayed about one month to see if hypercalcemia persists. Vascular supply to mediastinal gland may have been interrupted. Diagnosis should be reconfirmed. Contrast and PTH studies may be indicated.
7. **E** All symptomatic cases if unresponsive to medical therapy. This includes 4 mEq/liter calcium in dialysate, aluminum gels orally to bind phosphate, supplemental calcium and vitamin D to prevent hypocalcemia and hyperphosphatemia.
8. **C** In addition, if long-term follow-up is impossible, surgery should be considered.
9. **C** Generally accepted approach to probable hyperplasia.
10. **E** Blush on right side is either right parathyroid or right thyroid adenoma. Elevated PTH unilaterally suggests unilateral parathyroid process. Posterior ectopic location is usually superior parathyroid.

3. Head and Neck

INCIDENCE OF TUMORS

1. Five percent of all cancers
2. M > F
3. Older > Younger

HISTORY OF NECK MASSES ◀

1. > 7 years → congenital
2. > 7 months → neoplastic
3. > 7 days → inflammatory

ETIOLOGY

1. Chronic irritation; poor dental hygiene
2. Actinic rays—exposed areas
3. Tobacco ⎫ additive effect
4. Alcoholism ⎭
5. Culturally-defined
   a. Nasopharyngeal cancer—Orientals
   b. Hypopharyngeal cancers—Scandinavian women with Plummer-Vinson syndrome
6. Viral agents (?)—some correlation with antibody titers to Ebstein-Barr virus (nasopharyngeal) and herpes simplex (laryngeal)
7. Immune deficiency (cause or effect?)—response to DNCB correlates with extent of lesion and survival

DIAGNOSIS

1. Often late because of paucity of symptoms
2. Most discovered on careful physical examination
3. Check cervical lymph nodes systematically (See Fig. 3-1); all other nodes, liver and spleen
4. For leukoplakia, obtain "mouthwash" specimen for cytology
5. For mucosal lesions, topical toluidine blue may help delineate
6. Biopsy any suspicious area; plan biopsy so as not to interfere with subsequent

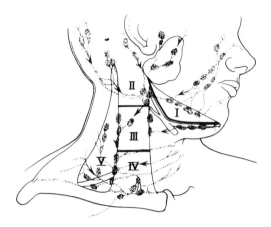

Figure 3-1 Lymphatic spread in head and neck cancer. *(From Gardner B, Polk HC, Stone HH, and Sugg WL (eds):* Basic Surgery. *Appleton-Century-Crofts, 1978, p. 184, with permission.)*

resection; best specimen obtained at border with normal area; positive biopsy is diagnostic, negative biopsy should be repeated
7. Routine bronchoscopy, esophagoscopy, laryngoscopy, and fiberoptic nasopharyngoscopy to rule out second primary
8. CT scan in selected cases to determine extent of tumor

STAGING

TNM

Tumor	T1	< 2 cm
	T2	2−4 cm
	T3	>4 cm
Nodes	N0	clinically negative
	N1	homolateral, mobile, < 3 cm
	N2	homolateral, single 3−6 cm or multiple < 6 cm
	N3	fixed or contralateral
Metastases	M0	no
	M1	yes

TREATMENT

General
1. Individualized, multidisciplinary approach, including surgery, radiotherapy, and chemotherapy as well as, in some cases, prosthodontic, psychiatric, and speech therapy and dietary instruction
2. Small lesions—local excision and/or radiation therapy
3. Larger lesions—resection in continuity with partial mandibulectomy, partial glossectomy, pharyngectomy, possible radical neck dissection (RND), and/or radiation and chemotherapy

Additional Treatment Methods
1. Radical neck dissection (RND) includes en-bloc *removal of*
   a. Deep cervical lymphatics and lymph nodes from mandible to clavicle, anterior midline to trapezius
   b. Sternocleidomastoid muscle, omohyoid muscle, internal jugular vein, occasionally spinal accessory nerve and/or thoracic duct
   c. *Preservation of* carotid artery, digastric muscle, vagus, phrenic, hypoglossal, and sympathetic nerves, brachial plexus
2. Radiotherapy—effective for treatment and palliation in many cases
3. Chemotherapy—including methotrexate, cis-platinum, Bleomycin
4. Immunotherapy—not widely used
   a. Specific—tumor-specific antigens given
   b. Nonspecific—BCG, corynebacterium, levamisole, or DNCB given to cause generalized immune enhancement
5. Cryotherapy
   a. Cold injury necrosis-involved tissues
   b. Painless rapid healing
   c. Best for localized lesions without positive nodes; especially for high surgical risk patients, or for palliation
6. Hyperthermia—thermal field of 44°C destroys malignant cells and increases radiation sensitivity; not commonly used

PROGNOSIS

1. Close lifetime follow-up essential for early detection and treatment of recurrence
2. Poor prognosis correlates with
   a. Anergy to DNCB
   b. Local blood vessel invasion on initial biopsy specimen
   c. Positive tissue culture from microscopically "tumor-free" surrounding areas
3. Overall prognosis varies with location and tumor type as well as stage:

Stage	Five-Year Survival (%)
Stage I (N0 T1)	77
Stage II (N0 T2)	67
Stage III (N0 T3 or N1 any T)	36
Stage IV (N2, N3 or M1)	9

SELECTED SPECIFIC SITES

Lip
1. 99 percent epidermoid
2. Usually arise at skin-vermilion border of lower lip
3. Two types: exophytic, endophytic

4. For localized lesion, surgical excision or radiotherapy is acceptable
5. Excellent prognosis

Buccal Musoca
1. 97 percent epidermoid
2. Three types: ulcerated, exophytic, or verrucous
3. Surgical excision with primary or flap closure
4. Radiation therapy is accepted alternative, except for well-differentiated or verrucous tumors
5. Prognosis—50 perecent five-year survival

Oral Tongue (mobile anterior two-thirds)
1. Small lesions—excision or radiotherapy acceptable
2. Large lesions—preoperative radiation, then excision
3. Because of high incidence of clinically undetected lymph node involvement, prophylactic RND advocated
4. Prognosis is best for tip of tongue lesions

Floor of Mouth
1. Usually epidermoid
2. Most involve nodes at time of diagnosis
3. Treatment is wide excision with in-continuity RND; occasionally preoperative radiotherapy is useful to shrink tumor
4. Overall five-year survival—50 percent

Base of Tongue (posterior one-third)
1. Usually early node involvement
2. Treated by radiation therapy or supraglottic laryngectomy
3. Prognosis poor—15 percent

Tonsil
1. Types
   a. Poorly differentiated epidermoid—75 percent
   b. Lymphosarcoma—15 percent
   c. Lymphoepithelioma—10 percent
2. Often mistaken for inflammatory lesion
3. Ipsilateral lymphadenopathy may be first sign; early distant metastases
4. Small lesion—radiotherapy
5. Large lesion—preoperative radiotherapy, then radical resection with RND
6. Overall five-year survival—60 percent

Nasopharynx
1. Types: Epidermoid, transitional cell, lymphoepithelioma, and others
2. Long delay in diagnosis common; then multiple symptoms possible:
   a. Nasal, aural, ocular, neurologic, olfactory
   b. Cervical lymphadenopathy
   c. Cranial nerve involvement (III–VII, IX–XII)

3. Surgically inaccessible; hence treated with radiotherapy
4. Complications of radiotherapy include:
   a. Dry mouth
   b. Epidermatitis
   c. Bone necrosis
   d. Pharyngitis
   e. Spinal cord myelitis
5. Prognosis poor; lymphosarcoma best; overall five-year survival—30 percent

Hypopharynx
1. Includes pyriform sinuses, aryepiglottic folds, lateral and posterior pharyngeal walls, postcricoid mucosa
2. Usually undifferentiated
3. Early metastases; diagnosed late
4. Lymphadenopathy or dysphagia may be first symptom
5. Treated by radical laryngectomy, hypopharyngectomy, RND or radiotherapy

Larynx
1. Type: squamous cell
2. Symptoms: voice change, hoarseness, odynophagia,"lump in throat"
3. Therapy
   a. In situ or suspicious epithelial lesion of true cord—strip entire epithelium
   b. Mobile glottic lesion—radiotherapy
   c. Fixed glottic lesion—total laryngectomy; if nodes involved, add RND and/or radiotherapy
   d. Supraglottic (usually diagnosed late)—if limited lesion in otherwise healthy patient, consider supraglottic laryngectomy
   e. Subglottic (rare)—laryngectomy and radiotherapy

Salivary Glands
1. Parotid (most common)
   a. Benign mixed tumor in 85 percent; the remainder will be mucoepidermoid or epidermoid cancer, adenocarcinoma, papillary cystadenoma lymphadenosum (Warthin's tumor), and others
   b. Treatment
      i. Expose entire gland
      ii. Excise superficial lobe (spare facial nerve, which runs between the lobes "like a fork through a hamburger")
      iii. Complete parotidectomy with sacrifice of facial nerve for invasive malignancy
      iv. Radiotherapy for recurrent or residual tumor
   c. Complications of parotidectomy
      i. Facial nerve paralysis or paresis
      ii. Frey's syndrome = gustatory sweating (etiology unknown)
2. Submandibular gland
   a. 50 percent malignant; most with lymphatic metastases
   b. Therapy: excision with RND

3. Minor salivary glands
   a. 75 percent malignant
   b. Therapy: excision; RND only if nodes involved

Solitary Neck Node with Unknown Primary

1. Complete head and neck workup
2. Blind biopsy of nasopharynx
3. Lung tomography
4. Upper gastrointestinal series
5. Intravenous pyelogram
6. Gallbladder work-up
7. If still no primary discovered, do RND; continue close follow-up until primary tumor appears

SELECTED BIBLIOGRAPHY

Attie JN, Sciubba JJ: Tumors of major and minor salivary glands: Clinical and pathologic features. Curr Probl Surg 18(2):1, February 1981
Woods JE, Beahrs OH: Head and neck surgery I. Surg Clin North Am 57(3):1, June 1977
Woods JE, Beahrs LH: Head and neck surgery II. Surg Clin North Am 57(4):1, August 1977

QUESTIONS

Directions: Each of the questions or incomplete statements below is followed by five suggested answers or completions. Select the *one* that is *best* in each case.

1. A 50-year-old male notices a painless, chronic ulceration of the floor of his mouth. There is no history of trauma and his oral hygiene appears good. He has smoked for 30 years. There is significant induration at the margins surrounding this 1-cm crater. The patient has been treated by another physician for the past month with a topical ointment, and the patient complains that the lesion has not changed. At this point, the diagnosis is best made by:
   A. Sputum cytology
   B. X-ray of the mandible
   C. Tomograms of the lesion
   D. Culture of the lesion
   E. Biopsy of the lesion
2. A 60-year-old male presents with a huge lobulated mass anterior to his left ear. It has been present for twenty years, slowly increasing in size. This history is characteristic of a:
   A. Cylindroma
   B. Mixed tumor
   C. Mucoepidermoid carcinoma
   D. Warthin's tumor
   E. Parotid adenocarcinoma

3. Cancer of the oral cavity is usually:
   A. Associated with drug abuse
   B. Squamous (epidermoid) in type
   C. Located on the hard palate
   D. Widely disseminated when first detected
   E. Diagnosed by excisional biopsy
4. A malignant posterior cervical node with no obvious primary lesion on oral or indirect laryngoscopic examination most likely arises from the:
   A. Gastrointestinal tract
   B. Central nervous system
   C. Lung
   D. Nasopharynx
   E. Scalp
5. Cervical lymph node involvement is *least* likely in localized cancer of the:
   A. Tongue
   B. Pyriform sinus
   C. Vocal cord
   D. Epiglottis
   E. Nasopharynx
6. Which of the following is *incorrect* concerning lingual thyroid in an 11-year-old girl?
   A. Is a congenital lesion
   B. Is best diagnosed by thyroid scan
   C. Requires needle biopsy for confirmation
   D. Often responds to thyroid hormone
   E. Rarely requires operation
7. Which of the following structures is generally preserved in a radical neck dissection?
   A. Sternomastoid muscle
   B. Submaxillary gland
   C. Omohyoid muscle
   D. Carotid artery
   E. Jugular vein
8. Radical resection of a malignant parotid tumor may require sacrifice of which nerve?
   A. Glossopharyngeal
   B. Hypoglossal
   C. Trigeminal
   D. Facial
   E. Nerve sacrifice is never indicated for parotid lesions
9. Which of the following is *least* likely to be true concerning cancer of the oral cavity?
   A. Squamous (epidermoid) in type
   B. Associated with poor oral hygiene
   C. Widely disseminated when first detected
   D. Diagnosed by incisional biopsy
   E. Located on the lip or lateral border of the mobile tongue

ANSWERS

1. **E** This is most likely a carcinoma, which must be biopsied because an early diagnosis is the only hope for cure. Over 90 percent of oral cancers are of the epidermoid type and commonly occur in patients who use tobacco or alcohol. The most frequent location of cancer of the oral cavity is the lateral border of the mobile tongue and the floor of the mouth immediately adjacent to the frenulum.

2. **B** This is a typical giant mixed tumor of the parotid. Excision without sacrifice of the facial nerve, if possible, is curative.

3. **B** Cancer of the oral cavity is usually epidermoid cell in type, detected in 45–85-year-old patients with poor oral hygiene, and who are cigarette smokers and/or alcoholics. It spreads locally rather than by hematogenous metastases and is best diagnosed by incisional biopsy. The most frequent location is the lip or lateral border of the mobile tongue and the floor of the mouth immediately adjacent to the frenulum.

4. **D** Nasopharyngeal cancer is notoriously difficult to diagnose and often requires blind biopsies.

5. **C** Being devoid of a submucosal lymphatic supply, the true vocal cords tend to have a low incidence of regional lymph node metastases until the cancer is far advanced. Hence, they respond well to either surgical or radiation therapy.

6. **C** A lingual thyroid is a congenital lesion representing failure of the thyroid anlage to descend in the neck from its point of origin in the base of the tongue. Diagnosis is by thyroid scan, which will reveal no thyroid tissue in its usual location. Treatment is with thyroid hormone suppression, which usually obviates the need for operation. Needle biopsy is contraindicated because it may result in bleeding and swelling of the lesion.

7. **D** A radical neck dissection is performed for the removal of metastatic disease in the cervical lymph nodes and includes, in addition, removal of the submaxillary gland, the sternomastoid muscle, omohyoid muscle, internal jugular vein, and even accessory nerve. The carotid artery is preserved under the thin skin flap and rupture of the carotid if infection occurs is a grave complication.

8. **D** The facial nerve passes through the parotid gland "like a fork through a hamburger." It separates the deep from the superficial lobe and may (although rarely) be sacrificed for a malignancy of the parotid gland.

9. **C** Cancer of the oral cavity is typically squamous, found in alcoholics or smokers with poor oral hygiene, diagnosed by incisional biopsy, and located on the lip, lateral border of the mobile tongue, or floor of the mouth adjacent to the frenulum. It spreads by local invasion rather than by hematogenous routes.

4. Adrenal and APUD System

ADRENAL

INCIDENCE

1. Benign nodules common
2. Carcinomas rare (0.2 percent of all cancer deaths)
3. M > F, average age is 44 for malignancies
4. Functional tumors—female predisposition
5. Virilizing tumors—usually children under 12
6. Cortical neoplasms usually benign; medullary neoplasms usually malignant
7. Of all adrenal malignancies, metastases most common

CLASSIFICATION

1. Functioning or nonfunctioning
2. Adenoma or carcinoma
3. Medullary neoplasms: neuroblastoma, pheochromocytoma, ganglioneuroma, mixed-type of ganglioneuroma
4. Adrenal cysts: endothelial cysts, pseudocysts, congenital glandular cysts, retention cysts, cystic adenoma
5. Other primary adrenal lesions: fibroma, myoma, lipoma, hemangioma, lymphangioma, fibrosarcoma
6. Cortical tumors
   a. Aldosterone-secreting—zona glomerulosa
   b. Corticosteroid-secreting—zona fasciculata
   c. Androgen-, estrogen-, progesterone-secreting—zona fasciculata and zona reticularis

DIAGNOSIS

1. Nonfunctional benign lesions—mostly discovered at autopsy
2. Malignant nonfunctional lesions—symptoms by progressive enlargement or metastatic disease
3. Stress or trauma may precipitate hemorrhage into an adrenal neoplasm or pseudocyst and lead to sudden adrenal insufficiency (apoplexy)

4. Uncomplicated lesion—effect of metabolic products. Diagnosis by measurement of metabolic products

LOCALIZATION

1. Calcification on plain abdominal x-ray
2. Intravenous pyelogram
3. Angiogram
4. Sonogram
5. CAT scan
6. Nephrotomogram

TREATMENT

1. Transabdominal exploration. If adrenal carcinoma is found, it is best resected as much as possible even if too advanced for cure. At times, adjacent organs (spleen, kidney, tail of pancreas) must be sacrificed
2. Metastatic disease—o,p-DDD (Lysodren); fractionated radiotherapy

METHOD OF ADRENALECTOMY

Anterior Approach
1. Allows thorough exploration for adrenal rests (in paraaortic area) or associated problems
2. Incision—midline or bilateral subcostal
3. *Left kidney*—open lesser sac, retract spleen superiorly and splenic flexure medially. *Right kidney*—divide hepatocolic ligament, retract omentum superiorly, retract right colon inferomedially, mobilize duodenum. Medial aspect of right gland partially obscured by inferior vena cava

Posterior Approach
1. Generally used in therapeutic adrenalectomy or to avoid transabdominal approach where exact diagnosis known preoperatively
2. Lessens postoperative paralytic ileus
3. Excellent exposure
4. Avoids peritoneal contamination if malignancy discovered
5. Method—prone jackknife position, symmetrical curvilinear incisions from tenth rib to iliac crest. Transect lumbodorsal fascia and pedicle attachments of the sacrospinalis muscle. Lyse pleura

COMPLICATIONS

1. Injury to adrenal veins—catastrophe avoided by careful, deliberate exposure and suture of such injuries

2. Pneumothorax (posterior approach)
3. Pancreatic injury, sepsis, pulmonary embolism (anterior approach)
4. Adrenal insufficiency (requires hydrocortisone 100 mg IV before anesthesia, during surgery, and every 6 to 8 hours thereafter)
5. Nelson's syndrome (pituitary tumors developing after adrenalectomy) occurs in 8 to 20 percent of patients after bilateral total adenalectomy—prevented by pituitary irradiation, even if this is not effective in alleviating Cushing's manifestations.
6. Mortality—2 to 3 percent

PROGNOSIS

1. Average survival after a diagnosis of adrenal carcinoma—two years
2. Metastatic disease—usually lung and liver, also bone, brain and skin
3. Local recurrence common

FUNCTIONAL TUMORS—HYPERCORTICOLISM

Etiology
1. Most common cause—therapeutic use of steroids
2. Excluding this, pituitary disease 63 percent, benign adrenocortical tumors 16 percent, malignant adrenocortical tumors 8 percent, and ectopic ACTH-producing lesions 13 percent

Diagnosis
1. Benign disease—insidious development of Cushing's manifestations
2. Malignancy—rapid course
3. Confirmation—plasma cortisol level, dexamethasone suppression test, ACTH or metyraprone stimulation test (See Fig.4-1)
4. Radiologic studies for localization—skull films to evaluate size of sella turcica, intravenous pyleography, nephrotomography, transfemoral adrenal venography, I-131 19-iodocholesterol adrenal scanning, grey scale ultrasonography
5. Adrenal venography—demonstrates small lesions, allows direct hormone level determinations, but intraadrenal hemorrhage or extravasation of contrast material is exquisitely painful, obscure later dissection, and may induce adrenal insufficiency

Treatment
1. Initial treatment of mild pituitary hypersecretion → pituitary irradiation; oral metopirone to control symptomatology during the course of radiotherapy
2. For microadenomas → transsphenoidal resection
3. More severe cases or recurrence after radiotherapy → bilateral total adrenalectomy (subtotal has been suggested but is debated)

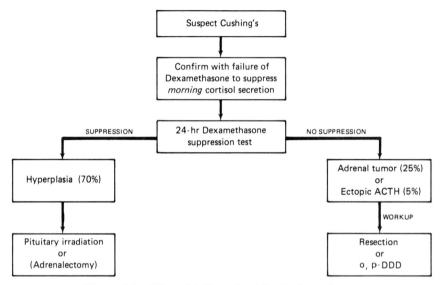

Figure 4-1   Differential diagnosis of Cushing's syndrome.

4. Cushing's syndrome → removal of offending lesion (either that producing ectopic ACTH or unilateral excision of the involved adrenal gland). Patients with inoperable or recurrent malignancy or those who cannot tolerate adrenalectomy receive o,p-DDD (Lysodren) → destroys cells of zona fasciculata of adrenal cortex; side effects include nausea, vomiting, lethargy, dizziness
5. Cyproheptadine (Periactin)—antiserotonin agent used in limited trial

PHEOCHROMOCYTOMA

Etiology
1. Adrenal medullary tumor (90 percent)
2. Other tissues of neural crest including organ of Zuckerkandl, celiac and mesenteric parasympathetic chain, renal hila, bladder neck, or mediastinum (10 percent)

Incidence
0.1 percent of routine autopsies, four times more common in autopsies of hypertensive patients

Diagnosis
Symptoms (in decreasing order of frequency)
1. Hypertension (90 percent): paroxysmal attacks or sustained hypertension
2. Headache (80 percent)
3. Excessive perspiration
4. Palpitation
5. Pallor
6. Nausea
7. Tremor
8. Weakness or exhaustion
9. Nervousness
10. Epigastric pain
11. Chest pain
12. Dyspnea
13. Flushing or warmth
14. Numbness or paresthesia
15. Blurring of vision
16. Tightness in throat
17. Dizziness or fainting

Confirmation of Diagnosis
1. Excessive catecholamine levels in plasma or urine—Most accurate is 24-hour urinary metanephrine excretion, as it is unaffected by diet and most drugs
2. Radiologic studies to localize tumor
   a. Plain abdominal x-ray, chest x-ray, grey scale ultrasound, IVP, nephrotomography, I-131 19-iodocholesterol scan
   b. Arteriography—requires close monitoring and adequate preparation with alpha-blocking agents, as provocation of sudden hypertensive crisis may occur

Medical Treatment
1. Alpha-blocking agents, sometimes beta-blockade as well
2. Fluid

Surgical Treatment
1. Anesthesia—enflurane
2. Fluid volume—Propranolol and phentolamine given prior to manipulation of tumor
3. Approach—transabdominal midline or transverse bilateral subcostal incision—7–10 percent are multiple and 10 percent are extraadrenal. Cholelithiasis is present in 1 of 4 patients
4. Procedure—completely excise involved adrenal together with surrounding adipose tissue (11 to 13 percent are malignant and proof of malignancy requires demonstration of local invasion or metastatic spread, as histologic criteria or the lesion alone are unreliable)
5. Bilateral—both adrenals are removed (one half are malignant versus 8 percent if solitary, 43 percent if extraadrenal)

Prognosis
1. Benign pheochromocytoma—96 percent five-year survival
2. Malignant pheochromocytoma—44 percent five-year survival
3. Extraadrenal malignancies—even worse prognosis

PRIMARY ALDOSTERONISM (CONN'S SYNDROME)

Etiology
1. Benign adenoma (80 percent)
2. Bilateral hyperplasia (20 percent)

▶ **Diagnosis (Six Ps)**
1. *P*ressure: hypertension
2. *P*otassium: low (sodium high)
3. *P*olyuria
4. *P*olydipsia
5. *P*aresthesias (due to metabolic alkalosis)
6. *P*eriodic muscle weakness

Treatment
1. Spironolactone and potassium to correct metabolic abnormalities
2. Operation

APUDOMAS

DEFINITION

"APUD" = cells which have a high *A*mine content, the capability of *A*mine *P*recursor *U*ptake and the enzyme *D*ecarboxylase

SITES

1. Neural crest of the hypothalamus
2. Pituitary → adenoma
3. Adrenal medulla → pheochromocytoma
4. Thyroid "C" cells → medullary carcinoma
5. Pancreas → islet cell neoplasms
6. GI tract → carcinoid tumors
7. Lung → oat cell carcinoma or carcinoid tumors
8. Parathyroid → hyperplasia or adenoma

PHYSIOLOGY

1. Excretory products of Apud cells are amines or polypeptides that are physiologically active:
   a. In general circulation (endocrine)

b. Only by direct contact with adjacent cells (paracrine)
2. Neoplastic change → apudomas

CLASSIFICATION

1. Orthoendocrine apudomas—secrete only their normal products (e.g., pancreatic islet cell tumors, pituitary tumors, thyroid medullary tumors, pheochromocytomas, carcinoid tumors)
2. Paraendocrine apudomas
   a. Secrete hormones characteristic of other endocrine glands (ACTH from a thyroid medullary tumor)
   b. Tumors of non-endocrine tissue giving rise to hormonal secretions (e.g., ADH from oat cell cancer of the lung)
3. Multiple endocrine adenopathies   ◄
   a. Wermer's syndrome (MEA I)—parathyroid, pancreatic, pituitary apudomas predominant, other glandular involvement less common
   b. Sipple's syndrome (MEA II)—adrenal medullary, thyroid medullary apudomas predominant. Parathyroid involvement (20 percent); submucosal lesions (MEA IIb). Treat pheochromocytoma *first*

INSULINOMA

1. Occurrence—fourth to sixth decade of life
2. Clinical findings—symptomatic fasting hypoglycemia, relief by glucose administration, and fasting blood sugar level under 50 mg percent *(Whipple's triad)*. In some, an insidiously developing organic brain syndrome due to neuroglycopenia is the only clue
3. Diagnosis—elevated fasting serum insulin level; however, false negatives require confirmatory testing
   a. Ratio of fasting immunoreactive insulin to serum glucose (IRI/G) > 0.3
   b. Stimulation of insulin secretion by intravenous tolbutamide
   c. Inhibition of insulin secretion by diazoxide
   d. 15-hour fast yielding blood sugar level after two hours of exercise < 50 mg percent—probably the most reliable test, but close observation is vital
   e. Malignant insulinomas—20 percent: mass lesion or common bile duct obstruction, elevated plasma human chorionic gonadotrophin
4. Localization
   a. Selective angiography (however, insulinomas are not associated with large vessel encasement or displacement and inflammatory changes in adjacent bowel, pancreatic pseudocyst, accessory spleens, or hyperplastic lymph nodes may be confusing; adenomatosis and very small lesions are not demonstrated)
   b. Transhepatic percutaneous portography with selective insulin assays
   c. Intraoperative mobilization of pancreas and careful palpation—most reliable means of localization

Other Islet Cell Apudomas

Apudoma	Presentation	Diagnosis	Treatment
Glucagonoma (alpha-2 cell)	1. Eczematoid or bullous dermatitis 2. Weight loss	1. Pancreatic mass 2. Diabetes mellitus 3. Serum glucagon	1. Local resection 2. Chemotherapy (often malignant)
1. Gastrinoma (Zollinger-Ellison syndrome)	Recurrent, severe and atypical peptic ulcer disease	1. High basal acid secretion 2. Serum gastrin > 600 pg/ml; calcium or secretin stimulation will more than double basal gastrin level 3. R/O Cowley's syndrome (antral G-cell hyperplasia) by gastroscopic biopsy	1. Cimetidine × 2 weeks, then 2. *Total Gastrectomy* (over 75 % malignant) 3. Palliation: streptozotocin and cimetidine
2. Somatostatinoma (non-beta cell-secreting VIP; however, prostaglandin E and F may be final common pathway)	Watery diarrhea [= pancreatic cholera; Verner-Morrison syndrome; WDHA (watery diarrhea, hypokalemia, achlorhydria) syndrome]; does *not* decrease even with cessation of oral intake	1. Hypokalemia 2. Acidosis 3. Achlorhydria	1. Fluid and electrolyte replacement 2. Local excision 3. Palliation: streptozotocin 4. Perhaps Indomethacin (75% of malignancies will have metastases)

5. Differential diagnosis—less than 50 percent of patients with Whipple's triad will prove to have insulinoma, the others will have
   a. Reactive hypoglycemia
   b. Hypoglycemia of pregnancy
   c. Addison's disease
   d. Cirrhosis
   e. Nonpancreatic tumors
   f. Factitious (self-induced) hypoglycemia
6. Management
   a. Bilateral subcostal incision
   b. Careful exploration for ectopic pancreatic tissue and liver for metastatic disease.
   c. Wide mobilization of pancreas and careful palpation
   d. Local resection *(enucleation)* of superficial tumor, if possible
   e. Deep lesion of body or tail, multiple lesions or no demonstrable lesion—*distal pancreatectomy*
   f. Clearly defined lesion in head that cannot be enucleated or on reexploration for persistent symptoms after distal pancreatectomy—*Pancreaticoduodenectomy*
   g. Serial intraoperative blood glucose levels to assess completeness of excision—should rise 30 mg percent per hour
7. Palliative management and prognosis
   a. Streptozotocin—for malignant insulinomas with symptomatic hepatic metastases
   b. Responders survive an average of three and one half years versus one and one-half years for nonresponders to this regimen
   c. Toxic reactions are common
   d. Other palliative drugs—Mithramycin, growth hormone, 7-deazaadenosine (tubercidin), alloxan, 5-fluorouracil

SELECTED BIBLIOGRAPHY

Harrison JH, Mahoney EM, Bennett AH: Tumors of the adrenal cortex. Cancer 32:1227–1235, 1973

Himathongkam T, Newmark SR, Greenfield MR, Dluhy RG: Pheochromocytoma. JAMA 230(12):1692–1693, 1974

Johnstone FRC: The surgical anatomy of the adrenal glands with particular reference to the suprarenal vein. Surg Clin North Am 44:1315–1325, 1964

Modlin IM: Endocrine tumors of the pancreas. SGO 149:751, 1979

Modlin IM, Stillman RM: Endocrine tumors. In Alfonso AE, Gardner B: Practice of Cancer Surgery. New York, Appleton-Century-Crofts, 1982, pp 351–378

Steinwald OP Jr, Doolas A, Southwick HW: Pheochromocytoma. Surg Clin North Am 49(1):87–98, 1969

QUESTIONS

1. A 46-year-old very hypertensive woman with polyuria and progressive weakness is found to have serum sodium of 148 mEq/L and potassium of 2.0 mEq/L. The most likely cause is:
   A. Carcinoid tumor
   B. Adrenal hyperplasia
   C. Adrenal carcinoma
   D. Pituitary tumor
   E. Single adrenal adenoma

2. You are called into the operating room by the gynecologists who are removing an ovarian cyst from a 32-year-old female. They have discovered a small mass superior to the left kidney and on palpation noted a marked increase in blood pressure. Your recommendation is to:
   A. Biopsy the mass and proceed based on frozen section diagnosis
   B. Perform a left adrenalectomy
   C. Perform a left nephrectomy
   D. Close the patient and reoperate only if she becomes symptomatic
   E. Close the patient and prepare for elective reoperation

3. A patient with cushingoid features is found to have elevated urine free cortisol and no suppression of plasma cortisol the morning after 1 mg of dexamethasone is given orally. Further studies reveal decreased plasma ACTH and no suppression of urine 17-hydroxycorticosteroids after the administration of 8 mg of dexamethasone given over 24 hours. The most likely cause of the problem is:
   A. Adrenal tumor
   B. Ectopic ACTH syndrome
   C. Pituitary tumor
   D. Idiopathic
   E. Pheochromocytoma

4. Elevated serum calcium is most likely to be associated with:
   A. Liver cell carcinoma
   B. Non-beta islet cell tumor of the pancreas
   C. Pheochromocytoma
   D. Oat cell carcinoma of the lung
   E. Carcinoma of the colon

5. Hypertension in a patient with a family history of medullary thyroid carcinoma is most likely the result of:
   A. Renal artery arteriosclerosis
   B. Renal artery fibromuscular hyperplasia
   C. Pheochromocytoma
   D. Glomerulonephritis
   E. Cushing's syndrome

ANSWERS

1. **E** The symptoms and signs suggest primary hyperaldosteronism; the most likely etiology is a single functioning adrenal adenoma.

2. **E** It is likely that the gynecologists have discovered a pheochromocytoma. A patient harboring a pheochromocytoma will have increased circulating levels of catecholamines. This will cause a chronic state of dehydration, resulting from excretion of fluid to compensate for the vasoconstriction. If the pheochromocytoma is removed during this operation, it is likely that the patient wil go into shock. Hence, the appropriate management is to complete the gynecologic procedure and close the patient. Afterwards a full work-up is performed while the patient is being treated with alpha- and beta-blocking agents, hydration, and careful observation. Elective resection of this tumor is performed at a later date.

3. **A** When hyperadrenocorticism is suspected, an overnight dexamethasone suppression test is the best first diagnostic study. One mg is given orally and will suppress ACTH secretion and, therefore, cortisol production in normal people, but not in patients with Cushing's disease or Cushing's syndrome. To differentiate adrenal tumor from ectopic ACTH syndrome from pituitary ACTH hypersecretion, a high-dose dexamethasone suppression test is performed and plasma ACTH levels are measured. Suppression of urinary 17-hydroxycorticosteroids to under 50 percent of baseline will occur with the administration of 8 mg of dexamethasone over a 24-hour period in patients with Cushing's disease (that is, pituitary hypersecretion). Plasma ACTH will be normal or elevated. In those with ectopic ACTH production, plasma ACTH is significantly elevated but there is no suppression with the overnight dexamethasone test. In patients with adrenal tumors, such as the one in question, the increased adrenal corticosteroid production will suppress ACTH secretion, causing a low plasma level, but there will be no suppression of urinary 17-hydroxycorticosteroids, even with high-dose dexamethasone.

4. **D** Hypercalcemia may occur with oat cell or squamous cell carcinoma of the lung. This is due to ectopic production of parathyroid hormone (pseudohyperparathyroidism).

5. **C** Multiple endocrine neoplasia type 11 describes a group of patients with a triad of inherited neoplasms including: (1) Medullary cancer of the thyroid, (2) pheochromocytoma, and (3) parathyroid hyperplasia. The occurrence of simultaneous medullary cancer of the thyroid and pheochromocytoma may result from a single defect in neural crest tissue of the APUD system. A high index of suspicion for this problem in patients having medullary thyroid cancer is necessary to avoid disastrous complications from unrecognized pheochromocytoma.

5. Lung

ANATOMY

Segmental Anatomy (See Fig. 5-1)
1. Right lung—three lobes, upper, middle, lower
2. Left lung—two lobes: upper and lower. Lingular portion on the left is the homologue of right middle lobe

Lymphatic Drainage
1. Right upper lobe → right paratracheal nodes
2. Right lower lobe → subcarinal → right paratracheal and posterior visceral
3. Right middle lobe → right paratracheal and subcarinal
4. Left upper lobe
   a. Upper portion → prevascular and left paratracheal
   b. Lower portion → left paratracheal
5. Left lower lobe
   a. Upper portion → subcarinal
   b. Lower portion → subcarinal and posterior visceral
6. Subcarinal nodes drain into right paratracheal nodes. Hence, *the right paratracheal nodes form the final lymphatic drainage pathway for the entire right lung and much of the left lung*

Blood Supply
1. Pulmonary arteries—carry deoxygenated blood from heart; parallel bronchi; supply lung parenchyma
2. Pulmonary veins—carry oxygenated blood to heart; run in interlobar septa
3. Bronchial arteries
   a. Arise from aorta and intercostal vessels
   b. Carry oxygenated blood to "servant" tissues
   c. Returns via peribronchial venous network to pulmonary veins
   d. Note that in normal lungs there are no actual bronchial veins

LUNG CANCER

ETIOLOGY

1. Cigarette smoking—evidence
   a. High correlation in human studies
   b. Proof of causation in animal studies

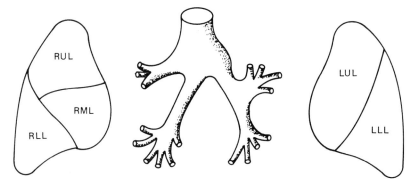

Figure 5-1 Bronchopulmonary segmental anatomy. Horizontal fissure separates RUL form RML, oblique fissure between RML and RLL, and oblique fissure between LUL and LLL. Lobes further divided into segments having individual branches of bronchi.

   c. Lung cancer increasing among women as smoking among women increases
2. Exposure to toxic agents
   a. Chromium
   b. Chloromethyl ether
   c. Radon gas

CLINICAL FINDINGS

1. Asymptomatic—average of three years between onset of lesion and symptoms
2. Cough—dry or productive
3. Dyspnea
4. Chest pain—shoulder pain with apical (Pancoast) tumor
5. Hemoptysis (almost all patients with hemoptysis have an identifiable underlying lesion)
6. Change of voice; hoarseness—involvement of recurrent laryngeal nerve
7. Wheezing, weight loss, fever, chills, clubbing of fingers or cyanosis
8. Hypertrophic pulmonary osteoarthropathy (symmetrical proliferative subperiosteal osteitis)—pain relieved after removal of tumor
9. Superior sulcus (Pancoast) tumor—shoulder and arm pain and Horner's syndrome
10. Hormonal manifestations
    a. Cushing's syndrome—ACTH usually from oat cell cancer
    b. Inappropriate antidiuretic hormone (IADH) secretion
       i. Usually fron adenocarcinoma or undifferentiated carcinoma
       ii. Results in severe hyponatremia, with confusion or coma
       iii. Treatment is fluid restriction

CLASSIFICATION (See Table 5–1)

Table 5-1   CLASSIFICATION OF PULMONARY NEOPLASMS

Type	Frequency among Primary Lung Malignancies	Overall 5-Year Survival	Comments
Squamous (epidermoid)	50%	24%	Keratin and epithelial pearls, intracellular bridges, 2/3 centrally located in large bronchi, closely associated with smoking, lymphatic mets may be hormonally active
Adenocarcinoma	20%	13%	Contain glandular elements, peripherally located, more common in females
Undifferentiated large cell	20%	14%	Peripherally located
Undifferentiated small cell or oat cell	9%	1%	Treated nonoperatively; may have neurosecretory granules with resultant Cushing's syndrome. Neuromyopathy. Brain mets common
Alveolar cell (bronchiolar)	1%	50%	Multicentric, peripheral, 2/3 resectable
Sarcomas	Rare	—	Radioresistant
Metastatic tumors	(30% of all patients with malignancy)	—	Sometimes resectable with BCG adjuvant therapy even if multiple, but primary must have been cured
Bronchial adenoma (malignant potential variable)	Rare	70%	1. Bronchial obstruction—recurrent pneumonia, hemoptysis 2. Classification a. Carcinoid—most common, radioresistant, centrally located, very vascular b. Adenoid cystic carcinoma (cylindroma) radiosensitive, commonly in trachea. c. Mucoepidermoid-pedunciated 3. Rx: usually lobectomy or pneumonectomy: bronchoscopic removal only in high-risk patients—recurrence common because of deep extension.

    c. Pseudohyperparathyroidism
      i. Usually from squamous cell cancer
      ii. Hypercalcemia with oat cell lesion is usually due to bone metastases
    d. Hypoglycemia
    e. Carcinoid syndrome
    f. Gynecomastia

DIAGNOSIS

1. Sputum examination—cytology or culture
2. Skin testing—tuberculin, histoplasmin, coccidioidin, recall antigens (test immunologic memory)
3. Chest x-ray and tomograms
   a. May show mass, infiltrate, pleural effusion, phrenic nerve paralysis, osteolytic bone lesions
   b. Solitary coin lesion is granuloma 55 percent, cancer 35 percent, hamartoma 7 percent
4. Lung scan: if scan shows defect larger than lesion itself, regional nodal involvement likely
5. Transpleural needle biopsy—especially for elderly patients who could not tolerate surgery
6. Bronchoscopy—with brushings or biopsies
7. Mediastinoscopy, mediastinotomy, scalene node biopsy, or open lung biopsy—provides the definitive diagnosis

Staging

TNM SYSTEM

TX	TO	TIS
Occult (i.e., secretions contain malignant cells, but no distinct tumor found	No evidence of primary tumor	In situ
T1	**T2**	**T3**
Less than 3 cm	Over 3 cm or involvement of visceral pleura, atelectasis or pneumonitis	Extension to parietal pleura, chest wall, diaphragm, mediastinum, main bronchus < 2 cm from trachea, or associated with atelectasis or pneumonitis of entire lung or pleural effusion
N0	**N1**	**N2**
Lymph nodes not involved	Positive regional lymph nodes	Positive mediastinal nodes
M0	**M1**	
No metastases	Metastases present	

Clinical staging

1. Occult = TX N0 M0
2. Stage I = TIS N0 M0, T1 N0 M0, T1 N1 M0 or T2 N0 M0
3. Stage II = T2 N1 M0
4. Stage III = T3 or N2 or M1

SURGICAL THERAPY

1. Thorocotomy and wedge resection of lesion, especially if lesion peripherally located and patient high risk for lobectomy →
2. Frozen section →
3. Lobectomy if localized to one lobe, or pneumonectomy if resectable but crosses into two lobes: must initially clamp pulmonary artery of tumor-bearing lung to determine if right heart can withstand the increased pressure load (especially in patients with long-standing obstructive lung disease and increased vascular markings)

► CONTRAINDICATIONS TO THORACOTOMY ("STOP IT!")

1. Scalene nodes positive for malignancy
2. Tracheal carina involved on bronchoscopy
3. Oat cell (undifferentiated small cell) → incurable
4. Pulmonary functions dangerously impaired: arterial $pCO_2 > 50$ is absolute contraindication. $FEV_1 < 1$ liter is relative contraindication. May improve with cessation of smoking, antibiotics, respiratory therapy
5. Infarction: recurrent myocardial infarction will occur in over one-third of patients undergoing general anesthesia three months following myocardial infarction; uncontrolled arrhythmias; angina pectoris with positive stress test rquires cardiac angiogram first
6. Tumor elsewhere: proof of metastatic disease

RELATIVE CONTRAINDICATIONS TO RESECTION

1. Involvement of phrenic nerve
2. Involvement of chest wall
3. Involvement of atrium or pericardium
4. Pancoast's tumor

COMPLICATIONS OF THORACOTOMY

1. Mortality—5 percent
2. Prolonged air leak—4 percent; most close spontaneously
3. Persistent collapse of remaining lobe—50 percent; most expand spontaneously
4. Empyema—7 percent; most drain via chest tube; occasionally decortication or thoracoplasty necessay
5. Cardiac arrhythmia—15 percent

ADJUVANT THERAPY

1. Postoperative megavoltage radiotherapy in Stage I or II lesion
2. Palliative radiotherapy in stage III, or emergently for SVC obstruction. Prophylactic brain radiotherapy for oat cell (?)
3. Chemotherapy: efficacy debated
4. Immunotherapy (BCG- or *Corynebacterium parvum*-induced); rationale: depressed immunity and depressed circulating T-lymphocyte levels are associated with poor survival

PROGNOSIS

1. Correlates best with extent of disease, *not* cell type except:
   a. Oat cell—worst prognosis
   b. Alveolar cell—fairly good prognosis

SELECTED BIBLIOGRAPHY

Harmon H, Fergus S, Cole FH: Pneumonectomy: Review of 351 cases. Ann Surg 183:719, 1976
Higgins GA, Shields TW, Keehn RJ: The solitary pulmonary nodule: Ten-year follow-up of Veterans Administration—Armed Forces cooperative study. Arch Surg 110:570, 1975
Margolese RG, Kreisman H, Wolkove N, et al.: Recent advances in management of lung cancer. Advan Surg 15:189, 1981
Wolfe WG: Noncardiac thoracic surgery. Surg Clin North Am 60(4):1, August 1980

QUESTIONS

DIRECTIONS: Each of the questions or incomplete statements below is followed by five suggested answers or completions. Select the *one* that is *best* in each case.

A 49-year-old male with a chronic cough is found to have a 2-cm coin lesion within the right upper lobe on chest x-ray.
1. Which of the following findings is *least* likely to be associated with malignancy?
   A. Dense lesion
   B. Cavitation
   C. Rounded lesion with umbilication
   D. Indistinct margins
   E. Heavy calcification

2. Of the following, the result *most* likely to permit nonoperative management of this patient is:
   A. Positive tuberculin skin test
   B. Negative sputum cytology
   C. Chest x-ray one year ago showing no change in size of lesion
   D. Negative bronchoscopy
   E. Negative percutaneous needle biopsy
3. Each of the following findings usually contraindicates thorocotomy *except:*
   A. Oat cells on bronchial brushings
   B. Resting arterial pCO_2 over 50
   C. Involvement of carina seen on bronchoscopy
   D. Scalene node positive for malignancy
   E. $FEV_1 = 1.0$ liter
4. If skin tests, bronchoscopy, and mediastinoscopy are negative, and pulmonary function tests are within normal limits, subsequent management should be:
   A. Trial of antituberculous therapy
   B. Thorocotomy and excisional biopsy
   C. Percutaneous needle biopsy
   D. Follow-up with yearly chest x-rays
   E. None of these
5. The most common pathologic type of lung cancer is:
   A. Epidermoid
   B. Undifferentiated large cell
   C. Oat cell
   D. Adenocarcinoma
   E. Bronchiolar carcinoma
6. Excluding oat cell cancer, the factor that correlates best with a five-year survival rate in lung cancer is:
   A. Blood vessel evasion
   B. Primary tumor size
   C. Lymph node involvement
   D. Segmental location
   E. Cell type
7. A solitary lung lesion found to be a metastatic tumor most likely arose from:
   A. Kidney
   B. Colon and rectum
   C. Brain
   D. Breast
   E. Skin
8. A 60-year-old male presents with tingling and pain in his left upper extremity radiating to the fourth and fifth fingers. On examinatioon you notice a drooping left eyelid and constricted pupil. These findings are best explained by:
   A. A subdural hematoma
   B. Scalenus anticus syndrome

    C. Cervical disk disease

    D. A Pancoast tumor

    E. Shoulder-hand syndrome

9. A 40-year-old male presents with hemoptysis. He is given codeine and placed on bedrest and the bleeding stops. Which of the following procedures should be performed at this time?

    A. Bronchogram

    B. Endotracheal intubation and ventilatory assistance

    C. Scalene node biopsy

    D. Bronchoscopy

    E. Thoracotomy

10. A 55-year-old man presents with coughing and hemoptysis. Chest x-ray and bronchoscopy confirm cancer. Which of the following findings absolutely contraindicates resection for cure?

    A. Phrenic nerve paralysis

    B. Extension to pericardium

    C. Positive mediastinal lymph nodes on mediastinoscopy

    D. Small cell (oat cell) undifferentiated cancer

    E. Calcification of mass

11. A 50-year-old male smoker with a known right upper lobe lung cancer presents with severe facial edema and a purple discoloration of the skin of the face and shoulders. He has blurred vision, a severe headache, nausea and vomiting. Upper extremity venous pressure is 50 cm water. Appropriate management is:

    A. Operative resection

    B. Venous thrombectomy

    C. Pericardiocentesis

    D. Radiation therapy

    E. Chest tube

DIRECTIONS: Each group of items below consists of four or five lettered headings or a diagram with five lettered components, followed by a list of numbered words or phrases. For *each* word or phrase, select the *one* lettered heading or lettered component that is most closely associated with it. Each lettered component may be selected once, more than once, or not at all.

    A Squamous cell carcinoma

    B Adenocarcinoma

    C Oat cell carcinoma

    D Bronchial adenoma

    E Bronchiolar carcinoma

---

12. Peripheral lesion which, although it usually is late to metastasize, is often multicentric in origin

13. The most common primary lung malignancy

14. Usually centrally located, slow-growing malignancy that has a 70 percent five-year survival rate after resection
15. Always treated nonoperatively

ANSWERS

1. **E** Heavy calcification is not characteristic of malignancy.
2. **C**
3. **E**
4. **B**
5. **A** Epidermoid carcinoma comprises 50 percent of the cell types of lung cancer. It is most common in men, occurs in the major bronchi, and spreads via lymphatics.
6. **C** The best correlation with five-year survival in lung cancer is with lymph node involvement. With the exception of oat cell, there are significant diffferences in five-year prognosis regardless of the cell type.
7. **B** Among solitary lung metastases, 30 percent originate from colon/rectum, 13 percent from breast, and 7 percent from kidney. In some cases, resection of the metastatic lesion may be curative—but only if the primary is cured, the metastatic disease is localized, and a long time period has elapsed between resection and the appearance of the metastatic lesion.
8. **D** A Pancoast tumor (carcinoma of the superior sulcus of the lung) will lead to Horner's syndrome and involvement of the brachial plexus.
9. **D** Prompt bronchoscopy must be undertaken at this point to determine the source of bleeding. There should still be enough blood present in the affected bronchus to allow this determination to be made.
10. **D** Oat cell cancer is treated with chemotherapy or radiotherapy and not resection. These are highly malignant tumors and comprise 20−35 percent of all lung cancers. The majority are centrally located.
11. **D** Superior vena caval obstruction syndrome is due to malignancy in 80−90 percent of cases, most commonly lung. Treatment is with diuretics, fluid restriction, and prompt radiation therapy. Anticoagulants or fibrinolytic agents may be used if thrombosis is occurring.
12. **E**
13. **A**
14. **D**
15. **C**

6. Mediastinum

ANATOMY

1. Anterior
   a. Thymus
   b. Ascending, transverse aorta
   c. Great vessels
   d. Trachea
   e. Lymph nodes and fatty tissue
   f. Any of these can give rise to an anterior mediastinal mass as well as any of the following: teratoma, goiter, pericardial or thymic cyst, Morgagni hernia
2. Middle
   a. Heart, pericardium
   b. Hila of lungs, tracheal bifurcation
   c. Phrenic nerves
   d. Lymph nodes and fatty tissue
   e. Other masses: cysts, pericardial, or bronchogenic
3. Posterior
   a. Esophagus
   b. Descending aorta
   c. Thoracic duct
   d. Nerves—vagus, sympathetic, intercostal
   e. Veins—azygous, hemiazygous
   f. Lymph nodes and fatty tissue
   g. Other masses—enteric or neurenteric cysts, hiatus hernia

CLINICAL FINDINGS

1. Respiratory—one half of patients
2. Asymptomatic—one third of patients
3. Chest pain
4. Weight loss
5. Dysphagia
6. Myasthenia gravis (thymoma)
7. Fever (intermittent with Hodgkin's disease)
8. Superior vena caval (SVC) obstruction
9. Malignancy—suggested by hoarseness, Horner's syndrome, severe pain, SVC obstruction

▶ DIAGNOSIS (The six Ss)

1. Symptoms
2. Site—chest x-ray especially lateral usually sufficient to determine anterior, middle or posterior mediastinum; fluoroscopy, tomography may be helpful; contrast studies of esophagus, bronchi, aorta, vena cava may be necessary
3. Scan—especially for thyroid
4. Sonogram—solid versus cystic
5. Scope—mediastinoscopy especially for sarcoidosis, lymphoma
6. Surgery—open biopsy is the definitive procedure; almost always necessary to rule out malignancy

Specific Disease Entities

1. Thymomas
   a. Adult
   b. Slow-growing
   c. Occur in anterior mediastinum
   d. Determination of malignancy is by gross tumor invasion, not by pathology
   e. Five-year survival if malignant—50 percent
   f. Associated with
      i. Myasthenia gravis in 50 percent (thymectomy helpful even if there is no thymoma—85 percent of patients with myasthenia gravis have normal thymus!)
      ii. Red cell hypoplasia
      iii. Hypogammaglobulinemia
2. Teratodermoids
   a. Young patient
   b. Calcification or teeth seen on x-ray
   c. May rupture
   d. 15 percent malignant
3. Neurogenic tumors
   a. Most common mediastinal tumors in all age groups (90 percent of posterior mediastinal tumors)
   b. Occur at costovertebral angle in posterior mediastinum
   c. Types
      i. Ganglioneuroma—from sympathetic chain
      ii. Neurofibroma—from intercostal nerves
      iii. Neurolemmoma—from intercostal nerves
      iv. Neuroblastoma—very malignant
   d. Malignancy—one half malignant in children, less than 10 percent malignant in adults
4. Pericardial (spring water) cysts—occur at cardiophrenic angles, especially on the right side. Resection if diagnosis is uncertain or for symptoms
5. Bronchogenic cysts—cause respiratory distress in infants, infection in adults
6. Enteric cysts—duplication of alimentary tract
7. Neurenteric cysts—in infancy associated with spinal column defects
8. Mediastinitis
   a. Acute—usually due to instrumentation, swallowed foreign body, trauma, leak of suture line, or postemetic rupture. Usually occurs in cervical

esophagus just below cricopharyngeus muscle. Treatment is broad spectrum antibiotics, fluids, oxygen, endoscopic removal of foreign body if perforation is small, surgical closure and drainage for continuing or significant leak (indications debated)
  b. Chronic—etiology is usually granulomatous infection of lymph nodes (usually histoplasmosis), fibrous mediastinitis (unknown etiology, late stages of fungal infections, especially histoplasmosis). Therapy is usually nonsurgical, but remove heavily calcified granulomas
9. Mediastinal emphysema
  a. Etiology—traumatic, iatrogenic, alveolar rupture
  b. Diagnosis—Hamman's sign (crunching sound on auscultation of precordium, produced by cardiac movement displacing air)
  c. Treatment—aimed at underlying cause

SELECTED BIBLIOGRAPHY

Burkell CC, Cross JM, Kent HP, Nanson EM: Mass Lesions of the Mediastinum. Chicago, Year Book Medical Publishers, 1969
Oldham HN: Mediastinal tumors and cysts. Ann Thoracic Surg 11(3):247, 1971
Stanford W, et al.: Mediastinoscopy: Its application in central versus peripheral thoracic lesions. Annals Thoracic Surg 19:121, 1975

QUESTIONS

DIRECTIONS: Each of the following questions or incomplete statements below is followed by five suggested answers or completions. Select the *one* that is *best* in each case.

1. A large mediastinal mass is discovered on a routine P-A chest x-ray. The next step is:
  A. Observe for one month and repeat x-ray
  B. Bronchoscopy
  C. Mediastinoscopy
  D. Esophagogram
  E. Lateral chest x-ray
2. The most common mediastinal neoplasm is:
  A. Thymoma
  B. Teratodermoid
  C. Pericardial cyst
  D. Enteric cyst
  E. Neurogenic
3. Aside from bronchogenic carcinoma, the most common cause of SVC obstruction is:
  A. Lymphoma
  B. Thyroid cancer
  C. Mediastinal fibrosis

   D. Malignant thymoma
   E. Traumatic
4. The most common cause of acute mediastinitis is:
   A. Esophageal rupture
   B. Surgery
   C. Extension from suppurative lymph nodes
   D. Extension from cervical infections
   E. Tuberculosis or fungal extension from lung involvement
5. Of the following, the structure that best demarcates anterior from posterior
   mediastinum is the:
   A. Sympathetic chain
   B. Thoracic duct
   C. Dorsal wall of trachea
   D. Dorsal wall of esophagus
   E. Posterior pericardium

DIRECTIONS: For *each* numbered word or phrase, select the *one* lettered
heading or lettered component that is most closely associated with it. Each
lettered heading or lettered component may be selected once, more than
once, or not at all.

   A   Thymoma
   B   Morgagni hernia
   C   Sliding hiatus hernia
   D   Pericardial cyst
   E   Ganglioneuroma

---

6. A lesion usually requiring operative intervention, commonly found in the
   posterior mediastinum
7. Anterior mediastinal lesion sometimes associated with red cell hypoplasia or
   hypogammaglobulinemia
8. Commonly found at right cardiophrenic angle and contains clear fluid

ANSWERS

1. **E**
2. **E**
3. **A**
4. **A**   in 60 percent of cases.
5. **C**   The anterior mediastinum is bounded by the posterior sternum, thoracic
           inlet, dorsal wall of the trachea, and the upward and backward projection
           of the anterior pericardial line.
6. **E**
7. **A**
8. **D**

7. Breast

INCIDENCE OF BREAST CANCER

1. Commonest cancer (except skin) in female—affects one in 14 women during lifetime
2. Female:male ratio = 100:1

RISK FACTORS

1. Previous cancer
2. Heredity (mother, grandmother, sister)
3. Nulliparity
4. Early menarche
5. Dysplasia (fibrocystic disease)
6. Cancer of uterine corpus
7. Endogenous hormones (theoretical)
8. Living in developed country
9. Oral contraceptives (?)
10. Reserpine (?)

PROTECTIVE FACTORS

1. Breast feeding
2. Oophorectomy early in life
3. Multiple pregnancies

CLINICAL FINDINGS

1. Usually painless lump (hence, self-examination important)
2. Also—the seven Ds
   a. Dermatological signs—erosion, eczema, Paget's disease of nipple
   b. Discharge—serous or bloody nipple discharge
   c. Depression—skin dimpling, nipple retraction
   d. Deviation—compare to other side
   e. Discoloration—pregnancy
   f. Discomfort—pain uncommon
   g. Dissemination—regional nodes, metastases to bone, liver, lung

DIAGNOSIS

1. *Bone scane* (Tc-99m) to screen for osseous metastases; then *bone survey* to confirm *absence of benign processes in suspicious areas* found on scan
2. *Xeroradiography*—most accurate radiographic study to help confirm breast cancer. Indications same as for mammography
3. *Mammography*—indictions:
    a. Evaluate opposite breast after cancer found on one side
    b. Evaluate ill-defined or questionable masses
    c. Work-up in metastasis from unknown primary
    d. Screening in high-risk patients
    e. Risk of induction of cancer due to radiation exposure precludes use in *routine* screening
4. *Biopsy*—*the* definitive procedure. Delay of up to about one week between biopsy of malignancy and mastecomy is probably *not* harmful

BENIGN LESIONS (80 percent of breast masses are benign)

1. Mammary dysplasia (fibrocystic disease)—commonest in 40−60-year group; increased risk of developing breast cancer
2. Fibroadenoma—well-circumscribed fibrous tumor, seen most commonly in 20−30-year age group
3. Duct ectasia
4. Intraductal papilloma—the most common cause of serous or bloody discharge. If not palpable or demonstrable on mammography, requires quadrantectomy of area from which discharge is expressed to rule out carcinoma
5. Fat necrosis—often secondary to trauma, but biopsy to rule out carcinoma
6. Acute mastitis—streptococcal or staphylococcal abscess, especially in lactating women. Early incision and debridement (often before fluctuant), to prevent progressive tissue necrosis, should be undertaken
7. Cystosarcoma phylloides—considered variant of fibroadenoma. Mastectomy only if malignant component
8. Cyst—may be treated by aspiration if it completely disappears and does not recur

CANCER

1. Location—usually in upper outer quadrant because that is where most of the breast tissue is located
2. Side—L > R by 5−10 percent (unknown why)
3. Nodes—histologically positive in 30 percent of those thought clinically negative
4. Staging (TNM)

T1	T2	T3	T4
< 2 cm	2-5 cm	> 5 cm	extension to skin or chest wall
N0	N1	N2	N3
no nodes	movable nodes	fixed nodes	supra- or infraclavicular nodes
M0	M1		
no metastases	metastases		

5. Treatment—Procedures available

	Removal of				
Type of Mastectomy	Breast	Axillary nodes	Pectoralis minor	Pectoralis major	Int. Mammary Nodes
Lumpectomy	no	no	no	no	no
Simple (total)	yes	no	no	no	no
Modified radical	yes	yes	yes/no	no	no
Radical	yes	yes	yes	yes	no
Extended radical	yes	yes	yes	yes	yes

Contraindications of Curative Mastectomy
1. Metastases
2. Grave local signs

Complications of Surgery
1. Injury to long thoracic nerve or brachial plexus
2. Necrosis of skin at suture line
3. Loss of split-thickness skin graft if used to close defect
4. Lymphedema of the arm—a rare complication of this is lymphangiosarcoma

Long-term Complications
1. Local recurrence
2. Metastases
3. Malignant pleural effusion
4. Hypercalcemia
5. Endocrine manipulation is more likely to be successful when tumor is positive for estrogen or progestin receptors (60 percent of tumors)

Therapy	Indications	% Remission
Estrogen	Postmenopausal	30%
Androgen	Premenopausal	20%
or		
Antiestrogen (Tamoxifen)		
Oophorectomy	Premenopausal	35%
Adrenalectomy	Recurrence after good response	30%
or	to oophorectomy (will ↓	
Hypophysectomy	estrogen level)	
Combined chemotherapy	Advanced stage	50-80%
Radiotherapy	Control of localized symptomatic	—
	mets (e.g., bone)	

PROGNOSIS

1. *Five-year survival:*
   a. Stage I (disease limited to breast)   85%
   b. Stage II (nodes involved)   66%
   c. Stage III (grave local signs)   41%
   d. Stage IV (metastases)   10%
2. *Other factors in prognosis:*
   a. Worse in male
   b. Bilateral involvement—50 percent in lobular carcinoma. (Hence, routine

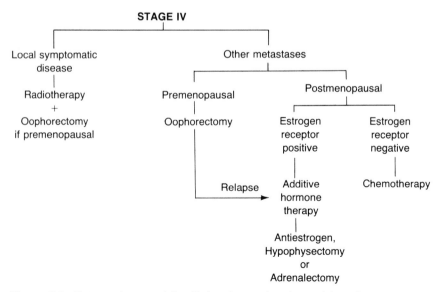

Figure 7-1   Pattern of sequential palliative therapy in advanced breast cancer.

biopsy of opposite breast for lobular carcinoma.) Overall 6 percent in breast cancer
c. Paget's disease of nipple has very poor prognosis
d. Pregnancy worsens prognosis and, hence, mastectomy should *not* await delivery
e. Inflammatory carcinoma has very poor prognosis
f. Medullary carcinoma is slow-growing with better prognosis

SELECTED BIBLIOGRAPHY

Cooperman AM, Esselstyn CB: Breast cancer. Surg Clin North Am 58(4):1, August 1978
Degenshein GA, Ceccarelli F, Bloom ND, Tobin EH: Hormone relationships in breast cancer: The role of receptor-binding proteins. Curr Probl Surg 16(6):1, June 1979
Schwartz SF: Evaluation of the patient with a breast tumor. Surg Clin North Am 53:717, 1973

QUESTIONS

DIRECTIONS: Each of the questions or incomplete statements below is followed by five suggested answers or completions. Select the *one* that is *best* in each case.

1. A 30-year-old female with serosanguinous nipple discharge is found to have no palpable breast mass. The most likely diagnosis is:
   A. Medullary carcinoma
   B. Intraductal papilloma
   C. Cystosarcoma phylloides
   D. Fibroadenoma
   E. Occult carcinoma
2. A 60-year-old female with a nine-month history of pruritis and eczema of the right nipple is found on needle biopsy to have clusters of Paget cells replacing the epidermis. No tumor or axillary node is palpable on either side. The most appropriate therapy is:
   A. Wedge excision of the upper outer quadrant
   B. Excision of the nipple
   C. Observation at monthly intervals
   D. Irradiation alone
   E. Mastectomy
3. A 60-year-old female presents with a 2.0-cm mass in her left breast. Frozen section shows replacement of breast fat by dense, myxomatous fibrous tissue with compression of intervening ductal epithelium. The most likely diagnosis is:
   A. Cystosarcoma phylloides
   B. Lobular carcinoma
   C. Fibrocystic mastopathy

     D. Mondor's disease

     E. Comedocarcinoma

4. Of the following, the greatest value of mammography is in:

     A. Differentiation of benign from malignant lesions

     B. Reduction of the need for biopsy

     C. Routine screening of all women of childbearing age

     D. Detection of nonpalpable masses

     E. Clinical staging of breast cancer

5. Curative mastectomy is probably futile in all of the following *except:*

     A. Breast cancer during pregnancy

     B. Extensive edema of the breast

     C. Ipsilateral arm edema

     D. Metastasis to the ribs

     E. Supraclavicular nodal metastasis

6. The most common location of a second primary breast tumor is:

     A. Upper outer quadrant

     B. Lower outer quadrant

     C. Upper inner quadrant

     D. Lower inner quadrant

     E. Periareolar

DIRECTIONS: For each of the questions or incomplete statements below, *one* or *more* of the answers or completions given is correct. Select:

     A   if only *1,2, and 3* are correct

     B   if only *1 and 3* are correct

     C   if only *2 and 4* are correct

     D   if only *4* is correct

     E   if *all* are correct

---

7. Which of the following is/are compatible with a T2 N2 M1 lesion?

     1. Tumor 1 cm in diameter

     2. Edema of ipsilateral arm

     3. Freely movable homolateral axillary nodes

     4. Malignant pleural effusion

8. Risk factors in the development of breast cancer include:

     1. Family history

     2. Uterine cancer

     3. Nulliparity

     4. Fibrocystic mastopathy

9. Associated with a higher risk of breast cancer:

     1. Unmarried

     2. Late menarche

     3. Residence in developed country

     4. Multiple pregnancies

10. Fibroadenoma:

     1. Multiple in 15 percent of cases

     2. Periodic variation in size is unusual

   3. Associated with excessive estrogen stimulation
   4. Commonly calcified
11. Mammographic indications of malignancy:
   1. Ill-defined margins
   2. Nipple retraction
   3. Focal calcification
   4. Increased translucency of breast tissue

DIRECTIONS: For *each* numbered word or phrase, select the *one* lettered heading or lettered component that is most closely associated with it. Each lettered heading or lettered component may be selected once, more than once, or not at all.

   A   Medullary carcinoma
   B   Intraductal papilloma
   C   Fibroadenoma
   D   Mammary carcinoma
   E   Paget's disease of the breast

---

12. Well-cricumscribed mass consisting of mammary duct cells compressed within proliferating fibrous tissue
13. "Grittiness" observed on biopsy specimen
14. Benign proliferation of epithelium lining large lactiferous intraareolar ducts
15. Nests of cells with clear cytoplasm and irregular hyperchromatic nuclei within a scaly, oozing nipple
16. Soft, fleshy, large but slow-growing tumor characterized by accumulation of lymphocytes around tumor cells

ANSWERS

1. **B**   Intraductal papilloma is likely, but cancer must be excluded by biopsy.
2. **E**   Paget's disease of the nipple is a highly malignant breast cancer.
3. **A**   Cystosarcoma phylloides is a variant of fibroadenoma but may at times have malignant components.
4. **D**
5. **A**   Breast cancer during pregnancy must be treated aggressively with early mastectomy.
6. **A**   Upper outer quadrant contains the majority of breast tissue and hence is the usual site of breast cancer, including second primaries.
7. **D**   12. **C**
8. **E**   13. **D**
9. **B**   14. **B**
10. **B**   15. **E**
11. **A**   16. **A**

8. Esophagus

GASTROESOPHAGEAL REFLUX AND HIATUS HERNIA

ANATOMY AND PHYSIOLOGY

Esophagus normally protected from acid by:
1. Lower esophageal sphincter
   a. Functional (not anatomical) sphincter
   b. Controlled by:
      i. Sphincteric smooth muscle
      ii. Autonomic innervation
      iii. Gastrointestinal hormones (especially gastrin)
   c. *Not* related to hiatus hernia
2. Secondary esophageal peristalsis
3. Bicarbonate-rich swallowed saliva (1000 to 1500 cc daily)

TYPES OF HIATUS HERNIA

1. Sliding
   a. Most common
   b. Cephalad migration of esophagogastric junction (EGJ) into the posterior mediastinum
   c. Anatomical abnormality due to:
      i. Increased intraabdominal pressure
      ii. Obesity
      iii. Weakness of ligaments and muscles
2. Paraesophageal
   a. Pouch of stomach herniates alongside esophagus
3. "Short" esophagus
   a. Usually due to long-standing esophagitis
   b. Congenital is exceedingly rare

CLINICAL FINDINGS

1. Dyspepsia
2. Regurgitation
3. Substernal burning pain
4. Bleeding
5. Stricture
6. Perforation (rare)
7. Pulmonary complications due to chronic aspiration

DIAGNOSIS

1. Upper gastrointestinal series (See Fig. 8-1)
2. Esophagoscopy
   a. To determine degree of esophagitis
   b. Biopsy may show
      i. Basal cell hyperplasia
      ii. Location of papillae close to endothelium
      iii. Inflammatory cells *not* necessarily seen
3. Bernstein test
   a. Perfuse distal esophagus with 0.1 N HC1
   b. Reproduces symptoms
   c. Differentiates from other causes of substernal pain
4. Esophageal pH probe test
5. Esophageal manometry and motility studies
   a. Demonstrates incompetent lower esophageal sphincter

MEDICAL THERAPY

1. Weight reduction
2. Avoid slouching, tight garments, large meals
3. Antacids
   a. Neutralize stomach content→
   b. Gastrin release→
   c. Increased sphincter tone
4. Elevate head of bed

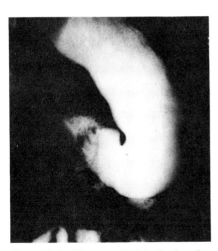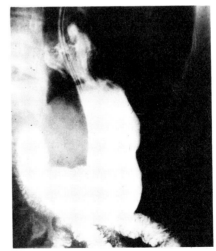

Figure 8-1 Upper gastrointestinal series with normal anatomy (left), and one showing sliding hiatus hernia (right).

   5. Avoid agents that reduce sphincter tone
     a. Fatty foods
     b. Chocolate
     c. Coffee
     d. Tobacco
     e. Alcohol
     f. Atropine
   6. Use of agents which increase sphincter tone
     a. Metoclopramide
     b. Prostaglandin F2 (experimental)

SURGICAL THERAPY

   1. Indications
     a. Failure of medical therapy (only 2.5 to 4 percent of patients are in this category)
     b. Peptic ulceration, stricture, hemorrhage, respiratory complications
     c. During laparotomy for concomitant disorders (commonly cholecystectomy)
     d. Paraesophageal hernia (all cases)
   2. Rationale
     a. Fixes EGJ below diaphragm where intraabdominal pressure elevates sphincteric pressure to reduce reflux (?)
     b. Construction of fundic compression valve surrounding lower esophageal sphincter
     c. Goal of operation is to restore EGJ competence
   3. Techniques
     a. Allison: repair crura of diaphragm and use phrenoesophageal membrane to maintain reduction, high incidence of recurrence
     b. Nissen: fundoplication—fundus wrapped around lower esophagus Probably most effective method, but complications include "gas-bloat syndrome" and dysphagia (See Fig. 8-2)
     c. Hill: posterior anchoring—GE junction to median arcuate ligament and preaortic fascia
     d. Belsey: Mark IV procedure—creates exaggerated esophagogastric angle to hold portion of esophagus in intraabdominal position. Does not work in severe reflux with stricture
     e. Collis: posterior gastropexy
     f. Vagotomy and pyloroplasty—performed in some cases to decrease acid hypersecretion
     g. Intraoperative manometry—may ↑ success rate of all accepted techniques
   4. Advantages of abdominal approaches
     a. Laparotomy is less painful
     b. Other intraabdominal organs can be examined
     c. Other intraabdominal pathology can be corrected
   5. Advantages of thoracic approaches
     a. Esophagus can be more completely evaluated

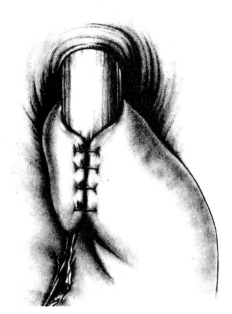

Figure 8-2 Technique of Nissen fundoplication *(From Maingot R (ed):* Abdominal Operations, *6th Edt. Appleton-Century-Crofts, 1974, p 1612, with permission.)*

   b. Resection can be performed if necessary
   c. Technically easier in obese patients

LATE COMPLICATIONS

1. Esophageal strictures due to reflux esophagitis
   a. Management
      i. Rule out malignancy
      ii. Esophageal dilatation
      iii. Repair of hiatus hernia (especially by Collis technique) with intraoperative dilatation via gastrotomy
      iv. Esophageal resection with colon interposition or gastric tube (rarely required)
2. Barrett's esophagus
   a. Pathology
      i. Extensive columnar metaplasia
      ii. Acquired condition due to chronic reflux
      iii. Premalignant (adenocarcinoma)
   b. Management
      i. Antireflux operation
      ii. Regular esophagoscopy to detect malignant change

3. Recurrent reflux esophagitis after surgery
   a. Etiology
      i. Usually due to technical error in initial procedure (15 percent failure rate)
   b. Management
      i. After multiple antireflux procedures and vagotomy/antrectomy, *duodenal diversion* may be performed
      ii. This diverts alkaline secretions (which may also cause esophagitis) via Roux-en-Y jejunal loop away from stomach

ESOPHAGEAL CANCER

ANATOMY

1. Arterial supply
   a. Upper—Inferior thyroid
   b. Thoracic—Bronchial arteries, aorta, and intercostals
   c. Lower—Left inferior phrenic, left gastric
2. Venous drainage
   a. Upper—variable
   b. Lower—coronary vein → portal vein
3. Histology
   a. Mucosa—stratified squamous epithelium and mucous glands
   b. Serosa—NON-EXISTENT, hence the two major problems with esophageal cancer:
      i. Early mediastinal spread
      ii. Anastomotic healing problems
4. Length from upper incisors to:
   a. Cricopharyngeus—15−20 cm
   b. Aortic arch—20−25 cm
   c. Inferior pulmonary vein—30−35 cm
   d. GE junction—40−45 cm

INCIDENCE

1. M > F
2. Age group 50−60 years

CLASSIFICATION

1. Carcinomas (mostly)
   a. GE junction—adenocarcinoma of gastric origin

b. Elsewhere—squamous cell of esophageal origin
2. Sarcomas
3. Carcinosarcomas

CLINICAL FINDINGS

1. Dysphagia—the first symptom; however, usually preceeded by at least a *year's* tumor growth
2. Severe weight loss
3. Weakness
4. Anemia

DIAGNOSIS

1. Gastrointestinal contrast series
   a. "Shelf"—irregular mass with horizontal upper border
   b. Annular constricting lesion
2. Esophagoscopy and biopsy—but *beware* of surrounding inflammatory tissue
3. Bronchoscopy—to rule out invasion of tracheobronchial tree

COMPLICATIONS

1. Bleeding—usually occult
2. Invasion of superior vena cava, aorta, trachea, bronchi, pericardium
3. Tracheoesophageal fistula—aspiration, lung abscess

TREATMENT

Surgical—only 30 percent will be resectable
1. Approach for resection
   a. Abdominal—to rule out metastatic disease, mobilize well-vascularized stomach, and perform pyloroplasty
   b. Then, thoracic—to perform high esophageal resection, then
      i. Esophagogastric anastomosis, or
      ii. Colon or small bowel interposition
2. Approaches for palliation _____
   a. Subcutaneous or substernal gastric bypass and radiotherapy of lesion
   b. Bougienage
   c. Intraluminal plastic tube

Radiotherapy
1. Especially for large tumors
2. May be used preoperatively to shrink tumor

PROGNOSIS

.1. Operative mortality—20 percent
2. Survival—5 percent at three years, somewhat better for GE junction lesions

SELECTED BIBLIOGRAPHY

Akiyama H: Surgery for carcinoma of the esophagus. Curr Probl Surg 17(2):1, February
    1980
Demeester TR, Johnson LF: The evaluation of objective measurements of gastroesophageal
    reflux and their contribution to patient management. Surg Clin North Am 56:39, 1976
Nemir, P, et al.: Diagnosis and surgical management of benign diseases of the esophagus.
    Curr Probl Surg 13(3): 1, 1976
Skinner DB, Demeester TR: Gastroesophageal reflux. Curr Probl Surg 13(1):1, 1976

QUESTIONS

A 50-year-old male presents with dyspepsia and substernal burning pain.
1. Assuming that UGI series confirms a sliding hiatus hernia, the Bernstein acid
   perfusion test would be helpful in:
   A. Confirming gastric hyperacidity
   B. Assessing tone of lower esophageal sphincter
   C. Assessing duration of reflux
   D. Differentiating other causes of substernal pain
   E. Proving "short esophagus"
2. Esophagoscopy will support the diagnosis of reflux esophagitis if biopsy
   shows:
   A. Basal cell hyperplasia
   B. Inflammatory cells
   C. Papillae close to endothelium
   D. Fibrosis
   E. All of these
3. The need for surgical intervention in this patient is best determined by:
   A. Duration of symptoms
   B. Size of hernia
   C. Amount and sequelae of reflux
   D. Sphincter tone
   E. Weight loss
4. The major goal of surgery if indicated for sliding hiatus hernia is:
   A. Closure of diaphragmatic defect
   B. Reduction of gastric acidity
   C. Resection of involved esophagus
   D. Relaxation of lower esophageal sphincter
   E. Restoration of esophagogastric junction competence
5. Adenocarcinoma of the distal esophagus and gastric cardia is best managed
   by:
   A. Feeding jejunostomy

  B. Radiation therapy
  C. Chemotherapy with 5-fluorouracil and Mitomycin-C
  D. Resectional surgery
  E. Colon bypass
6. A 65-year-old female develops difficulty swallowing that has been rapidly
   progressive over the past several weeks. Weight loss is marked and
   hematocrit is 30 percent. She denies heartburn. The most likely diagnosis is:
  A. Esophageal cancer
  B. Hiatal hernia with reflux
  C. Achalasia
  D. Cervical diverticulum
  E. Foreign body

ANSWERS

1. **D** Perfusion of distal esophagus with 0.1 N hydrochloric acid will reproduce
   pain and differentiate it from other causes of retrosternal pain such as
   angina pectoris. This is important because sliding hiatus hernia occurs in
   1 to 3 percent of routine upper GI series while only 8 percent will have
   symptomatic reflux. Hence, it may be an incidental finding in this patient.
2. **E** Although inflammatory cells and fibrosis are not essential in making the
   diagnosis.
3. **C** Indications for surgery include failure of medical therapy, peptic stricture,
   ulceration, hemorrhage, respiratory complications during laparotomy for
   concomitant conditions, and in all cases of paraesophageal hernia.
4. **E**
5. **D** Despite a poor prognosis, the best hope for survival in esophageal cancer
   is surgical resection.
6. **A** The most frequent cause of dysphagia in middle age and beyond is cancer
   of the esophagus. The next most common cause is stricture secondary to
   hiatal hernia, and then achalasia. Rapidly progressive symptoms with
   weight loss and anemia and the absence of heartburn suggest cancer,
   while a long history, with gradual onset of symptoms suggests benign
   causes. The diagnosis is confirmed by endoscopy and contrast
   radiography.

9. Stomach and Duodenum

PEPTIC ULCER DISEASE

ANATOMY (See Fig. 9-1)

1. Blood supply
   a. Lesser curvature
      i. (L) Gastric artery from celiac axis
      ii. (R) Gastric artery from hepatic artery
   b. Greater curvature
      i. (L) Gastroepiploic artery from splenic artery
      ii. (R) Gastroepiploic artery from gastroduodenal artery
   c. Fundus
      i. Vasa brevia from splenic and (L) gastroepiploic
   d. Duodenum
      i. Superior pancreaticoduodenal artery from gastroduodenal artery
      ii. Inferior pancreaticoduodenal artery from superior mesenteric artery
2. Lymphatic drainage
   a. Parallels arterial supply
3. Nerves
   a. (R) Vagus
      i. To posterior surface of stomach
      ii. Celiac plexus branch supplies GI tract to transverse colon
   b. (L) Vagus
      i. Anterior surface of stomach
      ii. Division through lesser omentum to liver
   c. Both vagal trunks send fibers (nerves of Latarjet) along lesser curvature to supply distal stomach

PHYSIOLOGY

1. Secretion
   a. Composition of gastric juice
      i. Volume: 500 to 1500 cc/day + 1000 cc/meal
      ii. Components:

Mucus	Glycoprotein, lubricant
Pepsinogen	From chief cells of oxyntic area
	Breaks peptide bonds at acid pH

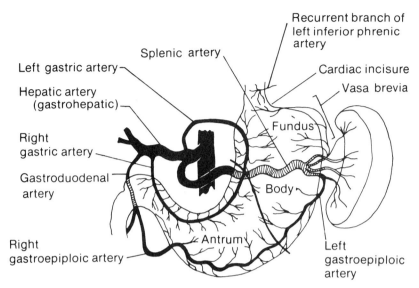

Figure 9-1 Anatomic divisions and blood supply of the stomach and duodenum.

Intrinsic factor	Mucoprotein
	Secreted by parietal cells
	Allows absorption of vitamin B_{12} in terminal ileum
Electrolytes	From parietal cells
	Potassium—5 to 10 mEq/liter
	$\left.\begin{array}{l} H^+ \\ Na^+ \end{array}\right\}$ + Cl^- —150 mEq/liter
Blood group antigens	Genetically determined trait occurring in about three fourths people
	Associated with decreased incidence of duodenal ulcer

b. Regulation of secretion
   i. Gastrin: from G cells of antrum and duodenum; in response to gastric distention and protein; stimulates acid, pepsin, gastric mucosal growth
   ii. Cholecystokinin-pancreozymin: from mucosa of small intestine; in response to fat, protein; stimulates gallbladder contraction, pancreatic enzyme secretion, and growth; inhibits gastric emptying
   iii. Secretin: from mucosa of duodenum/jejunum; in response to pH less than 4.5; stimulates pancreatic and biliary HCO secretion
   iv. Enterogastrone: from mucosa of small intestine; in response to fat; inhibits gastric acid secretion; existence postulated but never identified
   v. Bulbogastrone: from duodenal bulb; in response to acid; inhibits gastric acid secretion; existence postulated but never identified

   c. Stimulation of acid secretion
     i. Cephalic phase: brain → vagal efferents → parietal cells, chief cells, G cells
     ii. Gastric phase: food in stomach → gastrin from antral G cells → parietal cells, chief cells
     iii. Intestinal phase: food in small bowel → entero-oxyntin → parietal cells
   d. Inhibition of acid secretion:
     i. Acid chyme in duodenum → bulbogastrone → inhibits acid secretion
     ii. Fat within duodenum → gastric inhibitory peptide (GIP) → inhibits acid secretion and gastric motility
     iii. Feedback control of gastric emptying in response to osmolarity and pH
     iv. Antral pH less than 3 → inhibition of gastrin release
   e. Loss of mucosal barrier
     i. Reasons: shock or hemorrhage; alcohol; salicylates; bile salts, detergents
     ii. Results: acid enters submucosa → histamine released from mast cells → edema formation and more acid → intramural cholinergic fibers activated → pepsinogen secretion and muscular contraction

ETIOLOGY (debated)

1. Acid hyperesecretion due to psychic stress
2. Deficiency in production of enterogastrone
3. Decreased resistance of duodenal mucosa
4. Autodigestion by pepsin
5. Congenitally increased numbers of G cells and parietal cells
6. Blood group O and nonsecretors
7. Chronic diseases: liver, lung, pancreatitis

DIAGNOSIS

Clinical Findings
1. Epigastric pain relieved by food/antacids
2. Epigastric tenderness
▶ 3. Complications (bleeding, perforation, obstruction)
   a. "The restlessness of hemorrhage"
   b. "The stillness of peritonitis"
   c. "The writhings of colic"

Laboratory Studies
1. Normal or increased gastric acid
   a. Basal acid secretion (normal less than 1.5 mEq/hour)
   b. Maximally stimulated secretion (normal less than 20 mEq/hour)
     i. Histamine (hazardous)
     ii. Histalogue

    iii. Insulin (to test vagotomy)
    iv. Pentagastrin (experimental)
2. Serum gastrin level
    i. Normally 50 to 100 pg/ml
    ii. Suggestive of Zollinger-Ellison 200 to 600: try provocative test with secretin for diagnosis
    iii. Diagnostic of Z-E over 600
3. Test for occult blood in stool or gastric aspirate

Radiologic Studies
1. Upper gastrointestinal series (See Fig. 9-2)
    a. Distortion of duodenal bulb
    b. Eccentricity of pyloric channel
    c. Pseudodiverticulum formation
    d. Ulcer en face or in profile
2. Arteriography (for hemorrhage)
    a. Diagnosis of bleeding site
    b. Infusion of vasopressin
    c. Embolization of Gelfoam or clot
3. Upright chest or abdominal films. In perforation, free air is seen in 85 percent of cases (See Fig. 9-3)

Endoscopy (esophagogastroduodenoscopy)
1. To follow healing
2. With biopsy and cytology to R/O malignancy

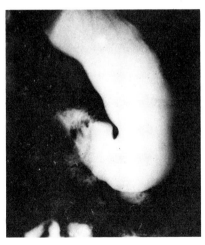 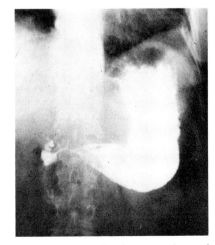

Figure 9-2 Normal upper gastrointestinal series (left) and one showing narrowing and severe scarring of severe duodenal ulcer disease (right).

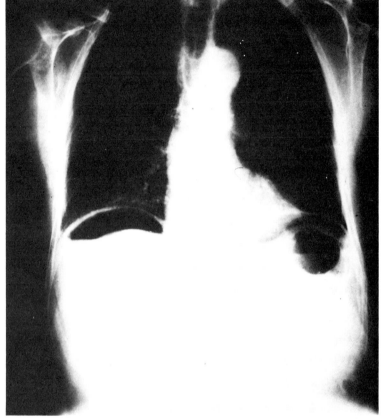

Figure 9-3   Upright plain film showing free subdiaphragmatic air. At laparotomy, a perforated duodenal ulcer was found.

3. In acute bleeding, 85 percent accurate (as opposed to 38 percent accuracy by emergency upper GI series)
4. For control of bleeding (experimental)

MEDICAL THERAPY

Aims
1. Relief of pain
2. Healing of ulcer
3. Prevention and control of complications

Diet
1. Bland diet (debated efficacy)

2. Frequent feedings and snacks
3. Avoid nicotine, steroids, reserpine, alcohol, salicylates, caffeine

Antacids
1. Hourly for active disease
2. One hour postprandial and at bedtime thereafter
3. Complications of antacids:
   a. High sodium content (Riopan is lowest)
   b. Constipation (Gelusil, Amphogel)
   c. Diarrhea (magnesium-containing antacids)
   d. Phosphate depletion
   e. "Milk-alkali" syndrome (absorbable such as sodium bicarbonate and calcium carbonate)
4. Preferred: Maalox, Mylanta, or Riopan

Pharmacotherapy
1. H_2 receptor antagonists
   a. Cimetidine
      i. Nonthiourea H_2 antagonist
      ii. 300 mg p.o. TID and HS
      iii. Parenterally for acute bleeding
   b. Metiamide: withdrawn due to agranulocytosis
2. Anticholinergics (example Propantheline): effectiveness debated
3. Sedatives
4. Experimental drugs
   a. Prostaglandins
   b. Bismuth compounds
   c. Pepsin inhibitors (sodium amylosulfate)

Gastric Irradiation
1. 2000 rads to parietal cell mucosa
2. Application is in elderly patients who are not surgical candidates

SURGICAL THERAPY

Indications
1. Unresponsiveness to medical therapy
2. Refractory hemorrhage
3. Obstruction
4. Perforation
5. Zollinger-Ellison syndrome

Procedures
1. Truncal vagotomy and drainage (pyloroplasty or gastrojejunostomy)
2. Selective vagotomy and drainage. Preserves vagal innervation to other viscera; hence, decreased incidence of diarrhea

3. Superselective (parietal cell) vagotomy. Spares visceral branches and nerves of Latarjet. Hence, no drainage procedure necessary, decreased incidence of diarrhea and dumping. Partial reinnervation may occur. Rare complication is localized avascular necrosis of lesser curvature
4. Antrectomy and vagotomy. Reconstruct with gastroduodenostomy (Bilroth I) or gastrojejunostomy (Bilroth II). BII may be antecolic or retrocolic. Low recurrence rate, higher mortality and morbidity than vagotomy/drainage
5. Subtotal gastrectomy. Remove antrum and parietal cell mass. Vagotomy not necessary
6. Gastrojejunostomy alone. Due to 20 percent recurrence rate, use only in very high-risk patients
7. Total gastrectomy. Only for Zollinger-Ellison syndrome or severe erosive gastritis
8. Omentopexy. For perforated ulcers. May be combined with vagatomy and pyloroplasty (See Fig. 9-4)

Complications
1. Of vagotomy
   a. Splenic rupture (avoid traction on greater curvature)
   b. Esophageal perforation (Levin tube should be used as guide in dissection)
   c. Periesophageal or mediastinal hemorrhage (clip vagi to prevent bleeding from accompanying vessels)
   d. Postvagotomy dysphagia (may require esophageal dilatation)
   e. Diarrhea, dumping (lessened by selective procedures)
   f. Incomplete vagotomy (intraoperative tests include Burge test, Grassi test, Lee's test, and Congo red test)
2. Of gastric resection
   a. Hemorrhage (usually responds to lavage and nasogastric suction, may require arteriographic control)
   b. Gastric retention (responds to NG suction)
   c. Duodenal stump dehiscence
      i. Most common cause of death after BII
      ii. Watch out for very inflamed duodenum
      iii. Drain if stump closure difficult
      iv. Occurs 3 to 6 days postoperatively
      v. Manifested by rigidity, fever, leukocytosis, hypotension
      vi. Therapy is immediate laparotomy, stump drainage, and management as high-output fistula. Do not attempt to close stump
   d. Anastomotic ulcer
      i. Etiology
         1) Too high acid initially
         2) Incomplete vagotomy
         3) Inadequate gastric resection
         4) Inadequate drainage procedure
         5) Retained antrum
         6) Zollinger-Ellison syndrome
         7) Too long afferent loop

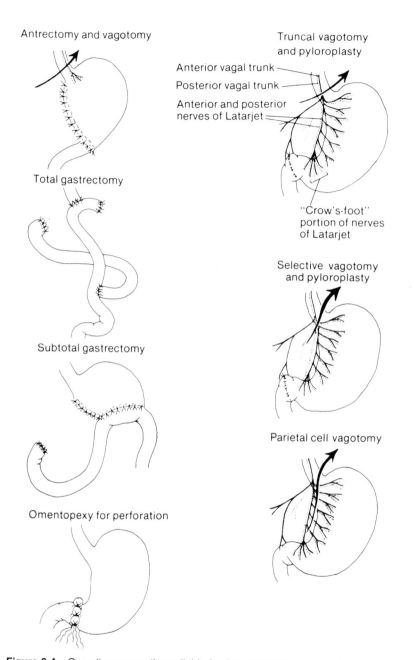

Antrectomy and vagotomy

Total gastrectomy

Subtotal gastrectomy

Omentopexy for perforation

Truncal vagotomy and pyloroplasty

Anterior vagal trunk

Posterior vagal trunk

Anterior and posterior nerves of Latarjet

"Crow's-foot" portion of nerves of Latarjet

Selective vagotomy and pyloroplasty

Parietal cell vagotomy

Figure 9-4   Operations currently available for the treatment of peptic ulcer disease.

     ii. Diagnosis
        1) Only 50 percent seen on GI series
        2) Diagnose by gastroscopy
        3) Gastrin level
        4) Hollander test (insulin stimulated acid output)
     iii. Treatment
        1) Complete vagotomy (possibly by transthoracic route)
        2) Adequate gastric resection
        3) Rarely responds to medical therapy
  e. Dumping syndrome
     i. Etiology
        1) Rapid entry of hypertonic fluid into duodenum or jejunum
     ii. Clinical findings
        1) Cardiovascular (palpitations, flushing)
        2) GI (vomiting, diarrhea, cramps)
        3) Occur shortly postprandial
     iii. Medical management
        1) Diet low in carbohydrates
        2) Fluid only between, not during, meals
        3) Anticholinergics (sometimes)
     iv. Surgical management
        1) Rarely required
        2) Interposition of antiperistaltic loop of jejunum
  f. Afferent loop syndrome (See Fig.9-5)
     i. Postprandial epigastric fullness
     ii. Relieved by vomiting bilious material
     iii. Food has already passed into efferent limb
  g. Efferent loop syndrome
     i. Postprandial epigastric fullness, pain
     ii. Relieved by immediate vomiting of food + bilious material
     iii. Treatment of loop syndromes
        1) Conversion to Bilroth I, or
        2) Tanner's Roux 19 reconstruction, or
        3) Braun's enteroenterostomy
  h. Anemia
     i. Iron deficiency (30 percent)
     ii. Vitamin B_{12} (megaloblastic)
  i. Alkaline gastritis
     i. Postprandial pain due to alkaline reflux
  j. Gastrojejunocolic or gastrocolic fistula
     i. Severe diarrhea and weight loss
     ii. Often preceded by symptoms of recurrent peptic ulcer disease
     iii. Effects due to adverse effects of colonic bacteria on stomach and jejunum
     iv. Requires surgical correction

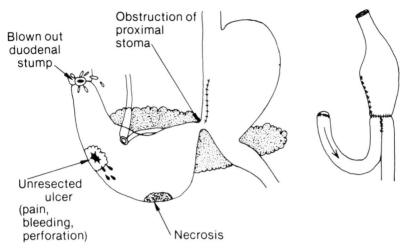

Figure 9-5 Sequelae (left) and management by enteroenterostomy (right) of afferent loop obstruction after a Bilroth II gastrectomy. *(From Artz CP and Hardy JD:* Management of Surgical Complications, *3rd Edt. W.B. Saunders Co., 1975, pp 452 and 454, with permission.)*

GASTRIC NEOPLASMS

INCIDENCE

1. Decreasing since 1930 (unknown why)
2. Still highest in Japan
3. M:F = 2:1; average age = 60
4. Positive family history—2 to 6 times the risk

CLASSIFICATION

1. Ulcerating—25 percent
2. Polypoid—25 percent
3. Superficial spreading—15 percent
4. Linnitus plastica—10 percent
5. Advanced—35 percent

PATHOLOGY

1. Adenocarcinoma—95 percent
2. Sarcoma, Lymphoma
3. Squamous cell (from esophagus)

▶ RISK FACTORS ("STOMACHS")

1. *S*pirits
2. *T*obacco
3. *O*rient—namely Japan
4. *M*egaloblastic (pernicious) anemia
5. *A*-blood group
6. *C*hronic gastric ulcer
7. *H*Cl—low (achlorhydria)
8. *S*ocioeconomic status—low

DIAGNOSIS

1. High index of suspicion in patients with:
    a. Vague epigastric complaints
    b. Anorexia (especially for meat)
    c. Weight loss
    d. Virchow's node
2. Gastric cytology will detect 72 percent
3. Gastroscopic biopsy—if inflammatory and not healed within three weeks of medical therapy, operation is indicated to rule out underlying malignancy
4. Upper GI series
5. Associated laboratory findings:
    a. Anemia—40 percent
    b. Increased CEA—65 percent
    c. Achlorhydria—20 percent

TREATMENT (DEBATED)

1. *Distal lesion*—radical subtotal gastrectomy, omentectomy, excision of celiac and hepatic lymph nodes. If spleen is removed, beware of necrosis of gastric remnant
2. *Proximal lesion*—proximal or total gastrectomy, splenectomy, nodes removed around tail of pancreas
3. *Gastroesophageal junction*—esophagogastrectomy
4. In any case, frozen section must confirm that resection margins are free of tumor

5. Reconstruction by gastrojejunostomy is preferred over gastroduodenostomy because:
   a. Technically easier
   b. Gastroduodenostomy more likely to be obstructed; recurrent disease
6. Other important considerations
   a. If significant weight loss, hyperalimentation is indicated for two weeks prior to operation
   b. Total gastrectomy performed only if *curative* because operative mortality is 12 perecent
   c. Lymph nodes dissection is not indicated in carcoma or lymphoma because hematogenous spread is as likely

PALLIATION

1. Bypass—preferably gastrojejunostomy
2. Resect bulky or bleeding lesion
3. Chemotherapy—especially methyl CCNU and 5-FU
4. Radiotherapy—for lymphoma especially

INDICATIONS FOR OPERATION IN GASTRIC ULCER

1. Radiologic or gastroscopic evidence of cancer
2. Histolog—fast achlorhydria
3. Positive cytology or positive biopsy
4. Chronic ulcer—does not show significant healing in three weeks, not completely healed in six weeks, or recurrent

CONTRAINDICATIONS TO EXPLORATION FOR ATTEMPTED CURE

1. Positive supraclavicular lymph node
2. Blumer's shelf, Krukenberg tumors (ovarian implants)
3. Umbilical mass
4. Malignant ascites
5. Other distant metastasis

PROGNOSIS

1. Overall five-year survival—5 to 15 percent
2. Better in cases with:
   a. Negative nodes (50 percent five-year survival)
   b. Carcoma or lymphoma

c. Superficial spreading cancer (90 percent)
3. *Early diagnosis is better than more extensive surgery in decreasing mortality rate*

GASTRIC POLYPS

1. Findings
   a. Anemia
   b. Achlorhydria (90 percent)
   c. Vitamin B_{12} deficiency (25 percent)
2. Treatment
   a. Small polyp—gastroscopic excision
   b. Large polyp—simple excision via gastrotomy or wedge resection
   c. Multiple (10 to 12) polyps—antrectomy plus excision of fundic lesions
   d. Benign polyps may be associated with cancer but are not themselves precancerous

MENETRIER'S DISEASE

1. A form of hypertrophic gastritis
2. Associated with achlorhydria, hypoproteinemia
3. Often misinterpreted as cancer

SELECTED BIBLIOGRAPHY

Buskin FL, Woodward ER: Postgastrectomy Syndromes. Philadelphia, Saunders, 1976
Cady B, Ramsden DA, Stein A, Haggitt RC: Gastric cancer: Contemporary aspects. Am J Surg 133:423, 1977
Cooperman AM (ed): Symposium on peptic ulcer disease. Surg Clin North Am 56:1231, December 1976
Dupont JB, Lee JR, Burton GR, Cohn I Jr: Adenocarcinoma of the stomach: Review of 1,497 cases. Cancer 41:491, 1978
Eisenberg MM: Physiologic approach to the surgical management of dudenal ulcer. Curr Probl Surg 14(1), 1977
Hallenbeck GA: The natural history of duodenal ulcer disease. Surg Clin North Am 56:1235, 1976
Ippoliti A, Walsh J: Newer concepts in the pathogenesis of peptic ulcer disease. Surg Clin North Am 56:1479, 1976
Johnson D, Goligher JC: Selective, highly selective, or truncal vagotomy? Surg Clin North Am 56:1313, 1976
Menguy R: Surgery of Peptic Ulcers. Philadelphia, Saunders, 1976
Ohme DO, et al.: Surgery for dudenal ulcer: A study relating indications to the results of surgery. Am J Surg 133:267, 1977
Passaro JE, et al.: Marginal ulcer: A guide to management. Surg Clin North Am 56:1435, 1976

QUESTIONS

DIRECTIONS: Each of the questions or incomplete statements below is followed by five suggested answers or completions. Select the *one* that is *best* in each case.

Five days after vagotomy and antrectomy for peptic ulcer disease, a 45-year-old male develops hypotension, fever, and severe epigastric and shoulder pain.

1. The most useful diagnostic study to identify the cause of this complication is:
    A. Serum amylase
    B. Electrocardiogram
    C. Gastroscopy
    D. Upper gastrointestinal series
    E. Upright abdominal and chest films
2. If subdiaphragmatic air is found on x-ray, the most likely cause is:
    A. Marginal ulcer with perforation
    B. Pancreatitis
    C. Gastrocolic fistula
    D. Esophageal perforation
    E. Blowout of the duodenal stump
3. Immediate therapy indicated for this complication is:
    A. Arteriography
    B. Exploratory thoracotomy
    C. Exploratory laparotomy
    D. Administration of H$_2$ blocker
    E. Observation and bed rest
4. Management of esophageal perforation during vagotomy should include:
    A. Nissen fundoplication
    B. Gastrostomy
    C. Jejunal serosal patch
    D. Simple two-layer closure
    E. Drainage alone
5. Parietal cell vagotomy is best performed in conjunction with:
    A. Pyloroplasty
    B. Gastrojejunostomy
    C. Antrectomy and gastroduodenostomy
    D. Antrectomy and gastrojejunostomy
    E. No other procedure
6. A 40-year-old female who is three days post-vagotomy and antrectomy develops a temperature of 105°F, hypotension, and leukocytosis, and blood culture grows *Serratia marcescens*. The most likely cause of this complication is:
    A. Duodenal stump disruption
    B. Subphrenic abscess

C. Atelectasis
D. Contaminated intravenous cannula
E. Pancreatitis
7. A 50-year-old female returns one year after vagotomy and antrectomy complaining of postprandial epigastric fullness that is relieved within 15 minutes by vomiting of bilious material. She notes that no food is found in the vomitus. The most likely cause of this problem is:
A. Dumping syndrome
B. Alkaline gastritis
C. Stomal ulcer
D. Afferent loop syndrome
E. Efferent loop syndrome
8. Palpitations, flushing, vomiting, and diarrhea and cramps occurring shortly after eating in a patient who has had gastrectomy and vagotomy are most likely due to:
A. Obstruction of afferent loop
B. Obstruction of efferent loop
C. Recurrent ulcer
D. Hypertonic fluid in small intestine
E. Incomplete vagotomy
9. Treatment of the condition described above includes:
A. Intravenous glucose
B. Insulin
C. Restriction of carbohydrates and fluid
D. Tanner's Roux 19 reconstruction
E. Enteroenterostomy
10. Diarrhea in gastrocolic fistula is due to:
A. Gastric acid irritating colonic mucosa
B. Pepsin-digesting colonic mucosal cells
C. "Blind loop" syndrome
D. Colonic bacteria entering stomach
E. None of these

DIRECTIONS: Each of the questions or incomplete statements below is followed by five suggested answers or completions. Select the correct answer(s). *All, some, or none may be correct.*

11. Cancer of the stomach:
A. Is increased in countries with high animal protein diet
B. Environmental factors are more significant than hereditary factors
C. Associated with blood group O
D. Associated with lower socioeconomic status
E. Incidence increasing in the United States
12. Gastric polyps:
A. If long-standing, are likely to undergo malignant degeneration
B. Occur as incidental findings in gastrectomy for cancer in about 30 percent of cases

    C. Associated with atrophic gastritis
    D. Associated with histamine—fast achlorhydria
    E. Commonest type is hypertrophic
13. Menetrier's disease:
    A. Is a form of hypertrophic gastritis
    B. Occurs with high basal acid secretion
    C. Associated with hypoproteinemia
    D. Often misinterpreted as cancer
    E. Associated with anemia

ANSWERS

1. **E**   Duodenal stump blowout will usually manifest as described x-ray shows free air.
2. **E**
3. **C**   Immediate laparotomy with drainage must be performed. No attempt should be made to completely close the duodenum at that time. The patient must then be treated for the resultant high-output small bowel fistula.
4. **D**   A simple closure will suffice. However, if the perforation is detected postoperatively, esophageal inflammation may make fundoplication necessary.
5. **E**   Due to sparing the nerves of Latarjet, gastric emptying remains normal, and hence no drainage procedure is necessary with highly selective vagotomy.
6. **D**   This is "third day surgical fever." See section on surgical infections.
7. **D**   The food has time to go into the efferent loop, while bile builds up in the obstructed afferent limb.
8. **D**   This is dumping syndrome caused by rapid entry of hypertonic fluid into small bowel.
9. **C**   Dietary therapy is usually successful; in rare cases, jejunal loop interposition will be necessary.
10. **D**   The treatment is surgical.
11. **B, D**
12. **B, C, D, E**
13. **A, C, D, E**

10. Gallbladder

CHOLELITHIASIS

ANATOMY

1. Common hepatic duct 3 to 4 cm long
2. Common duct
   a. 8 cm long × 6 mm diameter
   b. Enters duodenum at ampulla of Vater frequently joined by pancreatic duct
   c. Suprapancreatic, intrapancreatic, and intraduodenal portions
   d. Sphincter of Oddi surrounds CBD and pancreatic duct at papilla of Vater
3. Cystic artery
   a. Supplies gallbladder
   b. Arises from right hepatic (95 percent of cases)
4. Cystic duct about 4 cm long
5. Accessory hepatic ducts: may be missed and cause bile leakage
6. Many anatomic anomalies occur; in fact two-thirds of cases are anomalous

PHYSIOLOGY

1. Bile
   a. Volume: 250 to 1100 ml daily
   b. Stimulus
      i. Vagus
      ii. *Secretin* from duodenum (HC1 induced)
      iii. Bile salts
   c. Composition
      i. Lytes, proteins, cholesterol, fats, pigments
   d. Bile salts
      i. Cholic, deoxycholic, chenodeoxycholic acids
      ii. Conjugated with taurine or glycine
   e. Color
      i. *Bilirubin diglucuronide*
      ii. Arises from hemoglobin
      iii. Converted by intestinal flora into urobilinogen which may be reabsorbed
2. Gallbladder mucosa
   a. Secretion
      i. Mucus that allows passage of bile through cystic duct ("white bile")

ii. Calcium secreted in the presence of inflammation
b. Emptying of gallbladder
  i. Stimulated by *cholecystokinin* (arises from intestinal mucosa in response to fat in duodenum)

GALLSTONES

1. Composition
   a. Cholesterol
   b. Bile pigment
   c. Calcium
   d. Mixed (most common)
   e. Combined (layered)
2. Etiology (debated)
   a. Supersaturated bile leading to precipitation of cholesterol
   b. Infection
   c. Stasis
   d. Electrostatic factor
   e. Metabolic
   f. Obesity (fat, female, forty, flatulent, fertile)
   g. Diabetes: poor vascularity → early gangrene and perforation
   h. Cirrhosis

CLINICAL FINDINGS

1. Cystic duct obstruction
   a. Hydrops (palpable, tender gallbladder) → empyrea ("bag of pus")
2. Cholecystitis
   a. Fatty food intolerance
   b. RUQ pain
   c. Fever
   d. Nausea, vomiting
   e. Palpable gallbladder, if cystic duct obstruction
3. Emphysematous cholecystitis: gas-forming organisms
4. Acalculous cholecystitis—etiology
   a. Anatomic obstruction of cystic duct
   b. Ischemia of gallbladder
   c. Spasm of sphincter of Oddi
   d. Systemic disease or infection
5. Cholangitis
   a. Fever, shaking chills, jaundice (Charcot's triad)
   b. RUQ pain, shock, CNS depression
   c. Increased bilirubin, SGOT, alkaline phosphatase
   d. Amylase normal
6. Choledocholithiasis
   a. Incidence—12 percent in cholecystectomy
   b. Stones almost always from gallbladder

    c. Clinical course: common duct obstruction → dilated hepatic ducts →
       cirrhosis → cholangitis *(E. coli)* → hepatic abscesses
    d. Gallbladder usually not distended due to chronic inflammation
    e. Chemical abnormalities
       i. Increased bilirubin, alkaline phosphatase
       ii. Increased prothrombin time (due to decreased absorption of vitamin K,
          and promptly corrected by parenteral vitamin K)
7. Gallstone ileus
    a. Usually via cholecystoenteric fistula (usually duodenum)
    b. Usually obstructs at narrowest portion of small intestine (terminal ileum)
    c. Correct preoperative diagnosis rare, but can sometimes be made if air
       within biliary tract and intestinal obstruction coexist

DIAGNOSIS

1. Routine abdominal films
    a. 15 to 20 percent pickup
    b. Depends on calcium content of stones
2. Oral cholecystogram
    a. Uses 3 g oral Telopaque
    b. Nonvisualization may result from
       i. Failure to retain material
       ii. Poor absorption
       iii. Serum bilirubin over 1.8 mg percent
       iv. Loss of concentrating ability of gallbladder
       v. Faulty x-ray technique
    c. Repeat dose if first dose doesn't visualize
       i. *Only 2 percent* of gallbladders not visualizing at this study are found to
          be normal at laparotomy (See Fig. 10-1)
3. Intravenous cholangiogram (IVC)
    a. Applications
       i. Postcholecystectomy to evaluate ducts
       ii. If nonvisualizing oral cholecystogram
    b. Not reliable if serum bilirubin over 3.5 mg percent except in hemolytic
       jaundice
4. Percutaneous transhepatic cholangiography (PTC): requires dilated ducts
5. Endoscopic retrograde cholangiopancreatography (ERCP). Complications
     include pancreatitis, fever, hyperamylasemia, transmission of hepatitis
6. Sonogram—very accurate; especially useful in acute cases
7. Pipida scan—use in suspended acute cholecystitis; very accurate
8. Duodenal aspiration by peroral route; cholesterol crystals → gallbladder
     disease (rarely used)
9. Cholecystokinin-provocation test (rarely used)
    a. Causes RUQ pain mimicking previous attacks
    b. Use in cases of persistent symptoms in the face of normal x-ray studies

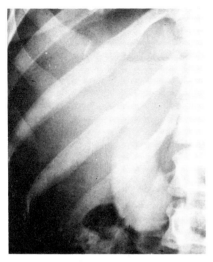 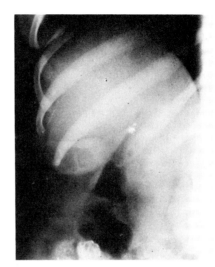

Figure 10-1 Normal oral cholecystogram (left) and one showing three large radiolucent gallstones (right).

MEDICAL THERAPY

1. Controversial
2. Oral chenodeoxycholic acid causes bile to become unsaturated
3. Relies on functioning gallbladder

DELAYED SURGICAL THERAPY

1. Risks of choledocholithiasis, empyema, gallstone ileus
2. Operative cancer mortality increases with age of patient

SURGICAL THERAPY

1. Cholecystectomy
   a. Watch out for right hepatic artery and common duct (See Fig. 10-2)
2. Cholecystostomy
   a. Drainage for distended gallbladder in poor-risk patients
   b. May use local anesthesia
   c. Will require cholecystectomy in two six months
3. Choledochotomy
   a. Indications to explore the common bile duct (CBD): ("OPEN IT") ◄
      i. Obvious reasons: palpable stones in CBD, dilated CBD, ascending cholangitis

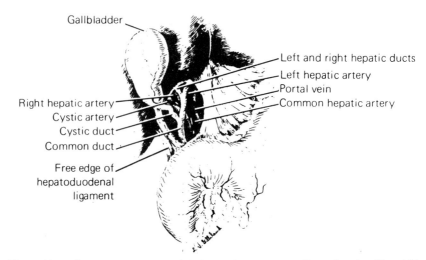

Figure 10-2   Structures encountered during cholecystectomy. *(From Dunphy JE and Way LW (eds):* Current Surgical Diagnosis and Treatment, *3rd Edt. Lange, 1977, p 526, with permission).*

    ii. Pancreatitis
    iii. Elevated bilirubin (jaundice)
    iv. No stones in gallbladder—only inflammation (relative indication)
    v. Intraoperative cholangiogram: shows stones in CBD (See Fig. 10-3)
    vi. Tiny stones in gallbladder (relative indication)
  b. Must leave T-tube for postoperative decompression for one week (spasm of sphincter of Oddi)
  c. Expect bilirubin to fall 1 mg percent daily for two weeks
4. Choledochoduodenostomy
  a. If all stones cannot be removed from common duct or in the case of primary common duct stones, especially in poor-risk patients who cannot tolerate further procedures
  b. Beware of missed carcinoma at ampulla!
5. Transduodenal choledochotomy with sphincterotomy
  a. For impacted stone at ampulla
  b. Allows biopsy to rule out malignancy

COMPLICATIONS

1. Overall mortality 1.8 percent
2. Abscess: subhepatic or subhrenic, bile leakage
3. Common bile duct stricture
4. Biliary cirrhosis

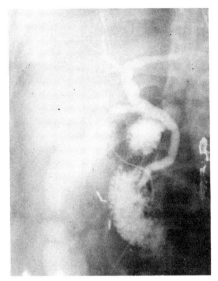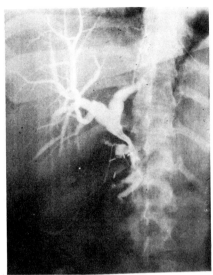

Figure 10-3   Intraoperative cholangiogram. Normal filling of common and hepatic ducts with good flow into duodenum (left) and one demonstrating a large stone in the common duct (right).

5. Pancreatitis
6. Postcholecystectomy syndrome: pain of unknown origin
7. Retained common duct stones
    a. Remove mechanically under fluoroscopic control
    b. Dissolve with saline or heparin infusions via T-tube
    c. Endoscopic transduodenal sphincterotomy
8. Persistant liver function abnormalities

CANCER OF THE GALLBLADDER

Pathology
1. Usually adenocarcinoma
2. 90 percent also have calculi

Diagnosis
1. Usually present in advanced stage
2. Sometimes discovered as incidental finding at cholecystectomy

Treatment
1. Wedge resection of galbladder and underlying liver, *and*
2. Excision of lymph nodes at hilum of liver
3. Right hepatectomy: no evidence that this increases survival and may actually increase mortality
4. No evidence that chemo- or radiotherapy beneficial

Prognosis—five-year survival
1. Overall—5 percent
2. If tumor recognized only by microscopic pathology with no involvement of muscularis propria—75 percent

Porcelain Gallbladder
1. Premalignant: requires cholecystectomy
2. *Polypoid lesions not* related to malignancy
3. *Adenomyomatosis:* normal variant, *not* premalignant

CANCER OF THE BILE DUCTS

Pathology
1. Usually adenocarcinoma
2. Tends to spread submucosally
3. Multicentric (?)

Clinical Findings
1. Jaundice

Diagnosis
1. Blood tests—extrahepatic obstruction
2. Visualized by PTC or ERCP

Treatment
1. Pre-op preparation with vitamin K to correct prothrombin time
2. Resection with wide margins; confirm by frozen section
3. May require Whipple procedure or hemihepatectomy
4. Palliative
   a. These tumors are usually slow-growing
   b. Dilate and place T-tube or U-tube through tumor, *or*
   c. Anastomose proximal duct to gastrointestinal tract over stent, *or*
   d. Percutaneous cannulation of proximal ducts

Prognosis
1. Distal duct tumor treated with Whipple—30 percent five-year survival
2. Others—dismal prognosis

SCLEROSING CHOLANGITIS

1. Associated with inflammatory bowel disease in 40 percent
2. Pathology is fibrous overgrowth—thickening of walls of bile ducts—narrow, beaded extrahepatic radicals, "stringlike" major ducts
3. Histologically difficult to differentiate from tumor
4. Treatment
   a. If extrahepatic with dilated intrahepatic ducts: hepaticojejunostomy or dilatation
   b. Steroids (?)
   c. If associated with inflammatory bowel disease, colectomy preventative (?)

SELECTED BIBLIOGRAPHY

Geenen JE, LoGuidice JA: Endoscopic sphincterotomy for diseases of the biliary tree. Adv Surg 14:31, 1980

Longmire WP Jr (ed): Symposium on gallstones. Adv Surg 10:61, 1976

Shaffer EA, Small DM: Gallstone disease: Pathogenesis and management. Curr Probl Surg 13(7):1, 1976

QUESTIONS

DIRECTIONS: Each of the questions or incomplete statements below is followed by five suggested answers or completions. Select the *one* that is *best* in each case.

1. A 25-year-old female with serum bilirubin of 10.5 mg percent, normal alkaline phosphatase, SGOT of 200 IU/ML and nonvisualizing double-dose oral cholecystogram most likely has:
   A. Serum hepatitis
   B. Cholelithiasis alone
   C. Cholelithiasis and choledocholithiasis
   D. Carcinoma of the head of the pancreas
   E. Pancreatitis
2. Postoperative Penrose drainage following routine cholecystectomy is justified most by the possibility of:
   A. Bleeding from the cystic artery
   B. Leakage from accessory hepatic ducts
   C. Prevention of adhesions to gallbladder bed
   D. Retained stones
   E. None of these
3. The most common vascular anomaly of the cystic artery is origin from:
   A. Left hepatic artery
   B. Common hepatic artery

    C. Inferior mesenteric artery
    D. Superior mesenteric artery
    E. Right hepatic artery with duplication

DIRECTIONS: For each of the questions or incomplete statements below, *one* or *more* of the answers or completions given is correct. Select:
  A if only 1, 2, *and* 3 are correct,
  B if only 1 *and* 3 are correct,
  C if only 2 *and* 4 are correct,
  D if only 4 is correct,
  E if all are correct

---

4. Elimination of retained common duct stones via T-tubes has been successful using:
    1. Protamine
    2. Bile acids
    3. Warfarin
    4. Ureteral basket
5. Suggestive of acute common duct obstruction:
    1. Total bilirubin = 11.5 mg percent (normal 0 to 1 mg percent)
    2. SGOT = 550 IU/ml (normal 10 to 50 IU/ml)
    3. Alkaline phosphatase = 450 IU/ml (normal 30 to 86 IU/ml)
    4. CPK = 500 IU/ml (normal less than 105 IU/ml)
6. Possible etiologies of acalculous cholecystitis include:
    1. Common channel
    2. Diabetes mellitus
    3. Parasitic infestation
    4. Anatomic obstruction of the cystic duct

ANSWERS

1. **A** Elevated SGOT is suggestive of hepatitis. The nonvisualizing oral cholecystogram was due to the elevated bilirubin.
2. **B** Accessory hepatic ducts from liver directly into gallbladder may be transected and leak bile postoperatively.
3. **E** Cystic artery arising from right hepatic artery with duplication is the most common anomaly.
4. **C** Saline irrigation has in some cases been sufficient, although use of bile acids and heparin has been reported. Ureteral basket passed with fluoroscopy can be used to remove stones through T-tube tract.
5. **B** Elevated alkaline phosphatase and bilirubin suggest common duct obstruction. In addition, serum cholesterol may be elevated. Elevation of SGOT and LDH imply prolonged jaundice or cholangitis.
6. **E** Also ischemia, collagen diseases, typhoid fever, antinomycosis. Incidence in United States is 5 to 10 percent of patients with gallbladder disease.

11. Liver

ANATOMY

1. Embryology—outpouching from duodenum
2. Size—2 percent of total body weight
3. Divisions—right and left lobes separated by imaginary line from gallbladder bed to vena cava. Further subdivisions (See Fig. 11-1)

BLOOD SUPPLY

Arterial
1. Celiac → common hepatic (gives off right gastric and gastroduodenal) → right and left hepatic
2. This comprises 25 percent of hepatic blood supply
3. Many anomalies

Portal
1. Portal vein—divides at porta hepatis into
   a. Right lobar—follows segmental ducts and arteries
   b. Left lobar—Transverse and umbilical portions
2. This comprises 75 percent of hepatic blood supply

Veins
1. Right, middle, left hepatic veins → vena cava
2. Accessory veins → vena cava

HEPATIC TUMORS

PATHOLOGY

Metastatic
1. Most common liver tumor is metastatic
2. Commonly from breast, lung, pancreas, etc.

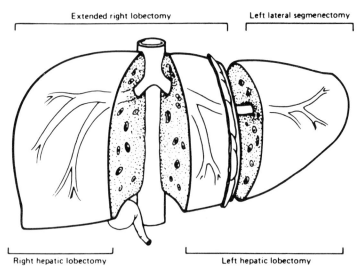

Figure 11-1   Hepatic resections: terminology. *(From Alsonso AE, Gardner B (eds):* The Practice of Cancer Surgery. *Appleton-Century-Crofts, 1982, p 244, with permission.)*

Primary
1. Uncommon in United States
2. Most have already metastasized when discovered (to hilar and celiac nodes, lung, peritoneum, veins)
3. Types
   a. Hepatoma—80 percent (hepatoblastoma in children)
   b. Cholangiocarcinoma—15 percent
   c. Hepatocholangioma—5 percent
4. Etiology
   a. Cirrhosis: postnecrotic, posthepatitic, alcoholic
   b. Clonorchis sinensis (Orient)
   c. Aflatoxins
   d. Vinyl chloride (angiosarcoma)

CLINICAL FINDINGS
1. Pain, distension
2. Weight loss, fatigue, anorexia, fever
3. Jaundice, hepatomegaly, mass, bruit, friction rub
4. Ascites, variceal bleeding, Budd-Chiari syndrome
5. Hepatic failure, intraabdominal bleeding

DIAGNOSIS

1. Scan—Tc-99m or CT scan
2. Arteriography—tumor usually supplied by hepatic artery, multiple tortuous vessels and blush → hepatoma
3. Alpha-feto protein—present in 80 percent of hepatomas
4. Laparoscopy and biopsy—must correct prothrombin time first with Vitamin K

TREATMENT

Resection—only 25 pecent are resectable (See Fig. 11-1)
1. Removal of up to 85 percent of a normal liver is compatible with life! This is because of prompt restorative hyperplasia which will often regenerate back to original mass
2. Occasionally metastatic lesions are resectable if localized to one lobe
3. Procedures may require thoracoabdominal incision

Transplantation
1. Experimental

Palliation
1. Intraarterial chemotherapy (FUDR)—implantable drug pump
2. Hepatic artery ligation—produces necrosis of tumor

POSTOPERATIVE COMPLICATIONS (OF MAJOR HEPATIC RESECTION)

1. Liver failure—inability to regenerate if extensive cirrhosis
2. Hypoglycemia
3. Hypoalbuminemia
4. Clotting factor deficiency
5. Right lower lobe atelectasis
6. Fever (common—often no etiology discovered)
7. Stress ulcers
8. Operative mortality—20 percent

Prognosis (average survival)
1. Primary hepatic tumor—6 months
2. Metastatic hepatic tumor—2 months

HEPATIC ABSCESS

Pathology
1. Solitary—usually right lobe, especially in diabetics; often curable
2. Multiple—both lobes, often incurable

Etiology
1. Direct spread from gallbladder
2. Portal spread from appendicitis or diverticulitis
3. Systemic spread from sepsis, subacute bacterial endocarditis, kidneys, lungs
4. Cryptogenic—in 15 percent, no etiologic source is found
5. Secondary bacterial infection in amebic, hydatid, or congenital cyst

Clinical Findings (often insidious)
1. Fever
2. Jaundice
3. Pain
4. Leukocytosis
5. Anemia

Diagnosis
1. Sonogram, scan, or CT
2. Arteriography

Treatment
1. Antibiotics based on culture and sensitivity—Metronidazole if amoeba suspected
2. Drainage or percutaneous aspiration—AVOID spillage into abdomen. If Echinococcus (hydatid), aspirate cyst content and replace with scolicidal agent prior to surgical manipulation.
3. Correct underlying etiology (biliary obstruction, etc.)

Prognosis: mortality rate
1. Multiple— 40 percent
2. Solitary—10 percent

BIBLIOGRAPHY

Balasegaram M: Management of hepatic abscess. Curr Probl Surg 18(5):1, May 1981
Calne, RY, Williams R: Liver transplantation. Curr Probl Surg 16(1):1, January 1979
Cooperman AM: Liver, spleen and pancreas. Surg. Clin North Am 61(1):1, February 1981
Madding GF, Kennedy PA: Symposium on hepatic surgery. Surg Clin North Am 57:1, 1977

QUESTIONS

1. Which of the following is *least* likely following a major hepatic resection in an otherwise normal patient:
   A. Increased prothrombin time
   B. Increased serum bilirubin
   C. Increased blood glucose
   D. Increased SGOT
   E. Decreased serum albumin
2. The *most* appropriate treatment for an amebic abscess of the liver is:
   A. Incision, drainage, and irrigation
   B. Excision
   C. Partial hepatectomy
   D. Metronidazole
   E. Observation alone
3. Which of the following hepatic lesions is associated with a lethal hypersensitivity reaction?
   A. Staphylococcal abscess   D. Hepatoma
   B. Amebic abscess   E. Hepatic adenoma
   C. Echinococcal cyst

ANSWERS

1. **C** When 50 percent or more of the liver is removed, the patient requires close monitoring and metabolic support for one to two weeks. Problems to be anticipated include hypoglycemia, hypoalbuminemia, coagulation abnormalities, hyperbilirubinemia, and sometimes elevated liver enzymes.
2. **D** Ten percent of the world's population harbors *Entamoeka histolytica.* In the intestine, this results in dysentery or colitis. From seeding via the portal vein, a hepatic abscess may supervene. This results in low-grade fever, leukocytosis, right upper quadrant tenderness, and characteristic x-ray or scan results. Differentiation from secondary infection with pyogenic organisms is difficult and may require percutaneous or laparoscopic needle aspiration. Upon diagnosis, metronidazole 750 mg orally three times daily for ten days is usually satisfactory. Very large abscesses may require percutaneous aspiration to prevent rupture, but operative excision of drainage is almost never necessary.
3. **C** The Echinococcus cyst is dangerous to the host for three reasons: (1) dissemination, (2) rupture with lethal hypersensitivity reaction, and (3) secondary bacterial infection. Hence, the goal in treatment is to remove the germinal lining of the cyst and the daughter cysts without spillage or implantation. The cavity is then treated with a scolicidal agent to destroy all remaining cysts. Preoperative preparation includes at least one week's treatment with an antihelminthic agent.

12. Portal Hypertension

ANATOMY

1. Hepatopedal
   a. Carry portal blood to liver if portal vein is obstructed but intrahepatic vasculature is normal
   b. Include: accessory veins of Sappey; deep cystic veins; epiploic veins; hepatocolic veins; hepatorenal veins; diaphragmatic veins; veins of suspensory ligament
2. Hepatofugal (See Fig. 12-1)
   a. More common. Circumvent blocked intrahepatic portal system
   b. Include
      i. Coronary vein → esophageal veins → azygos and hemiazygous veins → superior vena cava *(esophageal varices)*
      ii. Superior hemorrhoidal veins → middle and inferior hemorrhoidal veins → inferior vena cava *(internal hemorrhoids)*
      iii. Umbilical and paraumbilical veins → superficial veins of abdominal wall → superior and inferior epigastric veins *(caput medusae)*
      iv. Veins of Retzius (retroperitoneal) → inferior vena cava

Etiology
1. Presinusoidal portal hypertension
   a. Increased hepatopedal flow without obstruction
      i. Hepatic artery-to-portal vein fistula
      ii. Splenic arteriovenous fistula
      iii. Massive splenomegaly with increased flow in splenic vein
   b. Extrahepatic portal venous obstruction
      i. Developmental defects of portal vein
      ii. Cirrhosis causing portal vein thrombosis
      iii. Omphalitis with portal vein thrombosis
      iv. Sepsis with pylephlebitis
      v. Other causes of portal vein obstruction: trauma, severe enterocolitis, severe ECF depletion, blood dyscrasias, neoplasm, idiopathic
   c. Intrahepatic presinusoidal portal venous obstruction: schistosomiasis, myeloproliferative diseases, sarcoidosis, congenital hepatic fibrosis, arsenic toxicity, primary biliary cirrhosis, neoplasm
   d. Primary portal hypertension
2. Sinusoidal portal hypertension
   a. Alcoholic and nutritional cirrhosis
   b. Postnecrotic cirrhosis
   c. Biliary cirrhosis
      i. Secondary to gallbladder or large bile duct disease

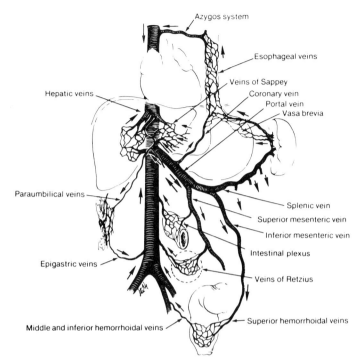

Figure 12-1 Hepatic portal collateral circulation. *(From Schwartz SI:* Surgical Diseases of the Liver. *McGraw-Hill, 1964, p 1199, with permission.)*

    d. Hemochromatosis
    e. Wilson's disease (hepatolenticular degeneration)
3. Postsinusoidal portal hypertension (Budd-Chiari syndrome = hepatic venous obstruction)
    a. Intrahepatic venous obstruction
      i. Acute alcoholic hepatitis
      ii. Oral contraceptives
    b. Extrahepatic venous obstruction: constrictive pericarditis, right heart failure, congenital membranous obstruction of the suprahepatic IVC, trauma, myeloproliferative disorders, primary or metastatic carcinoma of liver, kidney, or adrenal, oral contraceptives, pregnancy, sepsis, Jamaican venoocclusive disease (Bush Tea)

Most Common Cause of Portal Hypertension
1. *Cirrhosis,* which is intrahepatic presinusoidal, sinusoidal, *and* postsinusoidal
2. Microcirculation obstructed by: hepatic cell necrosis → hepatic fibrosis → *pressure from nodules of regenerating liver cells* → distortion and loss of sinusoids
3. Eventually about one third of portal blood flow is shunted intrahepatically through fibrous septa to hepatic venous radicles

CONSEQUENCES OF PORTAL HYPERTENSION

1. Esophagogastric varices
2. Encephalopathy; due to collateral circulation allowing intestinal metabolites (neurotoxins) to bypass detoxification in liver
3. Splenomegaly with hypersplenism
4. Ascites
5. Hepatorenal syndrome; due to decreased renal cortical blood flow

VARICEAL BLEEDING

DIAGNOSIS

1. History of varices
2. Signs of cirrhosis: splenomegaly (90 percent), ascites (frequent), hepatomegaly, jaundice, spider angiomata, hypoalbuminemia, prolonged prothrombin time
3. Esophagogastroscopy
   a. To rule out Mallory-Weiss tear, hemorrhagic gastritis, peptic ulcer disease
   b. To visualize varices
4. Upper gastrointestinal series. However, if both varices and peptic ulcer present, diagnosis of bleeding source will require other work-up
5. Measurement of portal pressure
   a. Normal portal pressure is less than 30 cm H_2O
   b. More significant is difference between free hepatic vein and wedged hepatic vein pressures (less than 4 normal, over 8 portal hypertension, over 20 bleeding varices)
   c. Techniques:
      i. Intraoperative cannulation of omental vein
      ii. Percutaneous occlusive catheterization of portal vein
      iii. Percutaneous splenic pulp pressure
      iv. Injection through dilated umbilical vein into left portal vein
      v. Selective superior mesenteric angiography for wedge pressure and venous phase to visualize varices

MEDICAL THERAPY

▶ If you suspect variceal bleeding, think "VARICEAL":
1. Volume: intravenous fluid and blood
2. Assess: look for overt signs of cirrhosis; endoscope to confirm that varices are indeed source of bleeding; if so, consider endoscopic sclerotherapy
3. Reach for the Sengstaken-Blakemore triple lumen tube; esophageal and gastric balloons, lumen for gastric aspiration; hazards include aspiration

pneumonia, esophageal rupture, respiratory obstruction if balloon slips into pharynx
4. *I*nfuse vasopression (Pitressin) → sphlanchnic vasoconstriction → reduced portal blood flow; dose is 0.5 units per minute for one hour via peripheral vein
5. *C*oags: reverse coagulation abnormalities with vitamin K and fresh frozen plasma
6. *E*ncephalopathy: decrease formation and absorption of ammonia with gastric lavage, colonic washout and oral nonabsorbable antibiotics
7. *A*ngiography: especially hepatic vein cannulation to measure wedged hepatic vein pressure
8. *L*ast resort: operate

SURGICAL THERAPY

1. Indications
   a. Failure of medical therapy during acute bleed
   b. Previous bleed
   c. Prophylactically in patients with varices (30 percent will bleed within five years)—debated
2. Procedures
   a. During acute bleed
      i. Mesocaval H-graft; rapid procedure using Dacron graft
      ii. Portacaval shunt; high mortality (50 percent)
      iii. Variceal ligation; rapid control of bleeding, but rebleeding frequent
      iv. Subcardiac porto-azygous disconnection (Tanner procedure); rebleeding frequent
   b. Elective portal decompression (See Fig. 12-2)

Procedure	Technique	Problems		Advantages	
End-to-side portacaval	Portal vein transected and anastomosed to side of IVC	i.	Hepatic artery cannot completely compensate for loss of portal flow Encephalopathy		When combined with arterialization of hepatic stump of portal vein may decrease encephalopathy
Side-to-side portacaval	Anastomose side-to-side in situ, or mesocaval, mesorenal, or central splenorenal (Provides continuity between	i.	Hepatic limb flow is usually retrograde, which further increases encephalopathy	i. ii.	Decompresses intrahepatic portal venous system in Budd-Chiari syndrome or with ascites Mesocaval H-graft is simple and rapid

(continued)

Procedure	Technique	Problems	Advantages
	hepatic side of portal vein and portal system)		
Distal splenorenal (Warren)	Splenic end of transected splenic vein anastomosed to side of renal vein; coronary vein tied	i. Technically difficult ii. Portal flow not totally diverted from liver	i. Less encephalopathy

PROGNOSIS

1. Bleeding stopped without surgery—60 percent
2. Emergency surgery necessary—25 percent (varies)
3. Death due to hemorrhage—15 percent
4. Mortality in elective shunt—5 to 10 percent
5. Elective shunt is preferable to emergency shunt because patient may be prepared and thus switched into a more favorable Child's category

Criteria for Favorable Prognosis (Child's Classification)

	Class A	Class B	Class C
Bilirubin	<2.0	2.0-3.0	>3.0
Albumin	>3.5	3.0-3.5	<3.0
Ascites	None	Minimal	Severe
Encephalopathy	None	Minimal	Severe
Nutritional impairment	None	Minimal	Severe

ASCITES

PATHOGENESIS

1. Redistribution of fluid between plasma and extravascular fluid
   a. Hypoalbuminemia, resulting from
      i. Decreased hepatic synthesis
      ii. Increased plasma volume
   b. Portal vein and hepatic sinusoidal hypertension
      i. Hydrostatic pressure in hepatic sinusoids and splanchnic capillaries and lymphatics due to portal hypertension
      ii. Ascitic fluid leaks from suface of liver and through serosal surface of mesentery and intestines
2. Excessive salt and water retention by the kidney, due to
   a. Loss of fluid as ascites → decreased effective extracellular fluid →

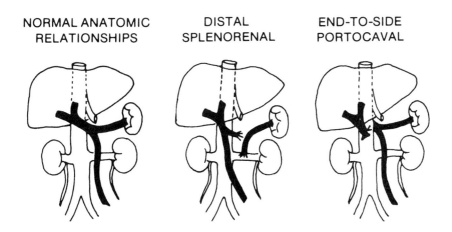

FUNCTIONAL SIDE-TO-SIDE PORTOCAVAL

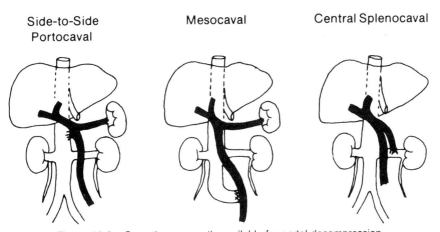

Figure 12-2 Operations currently available for portal decompression.

decreased renal artery blood flow → salt and water retention → increased intravascular hydrostatic pressure and decreased plasma oncotic pressure → more ascites
b. Redistribution of intrarenal blood flow of unknown mechanism
c. Decreased third factor
d. Increased aldosterone effects
3. Thoracic duct capacity exceeded (normally, the thoracic duct lymph drains some ascitic fluid)

MEDICAL THERAPY

Key is to induce spontaneous sodium diuresis
1. Rigid sodium restriction (250 mg salt daily)
2. Fluid restriction (1500 ml daily)

    a. KC1 for resultant hypokalemia

    b. Further salt and water restriction for hyponatremia (unless sodium under 125 mEq/liter)

3. Diuretics

    a. Indications

        i. Salt and water restriction alone not adequate, or

        ii. Urine sodium less than 10 mEq daily despite above

    b. Complication: dangerous decrease in plasma volume especially in patients with ascites but without peripheral edema

4. Paracentesis: diagnostic or therapeutic for: respiratory problems or imminent rupture of umbilicus

5. Intravenous albumin—probably ineffective

SURGICAL THERAPY

1. LeVeen or Denver shunt

    a. Method—peritoneojugular shunt using a subcutaneous silicone tube with a *pressure-activated* one-way valve. Excessive rise of CVP closes valve to prevent fluid overload (See Fig. 12-3)

    b. Concomitant therapy

        i. Abdominal elastic binder

        ii. Furosemide for 10 days postoperatively

        iii. Respiratory exercises

    c. The aim is to increase mobilization and excretion of ascitic fluid and encourage continued flow through valve. Vigorous medical therapy must be terminated postoperatively to maintain flow in order to keep valve patent

2. Portacaval shunt

    a. Very high mortality, no longer recommended for ascites

SELECTED BIBLIOGRAPHY

Child CG III: Portal Hypertension. Philadelphia, Saunders, 1974

Leveen HH, Wapnick S, Diaz C, et al.: Ascites—its correction by peritoneovenous shunting. Curr Probl Surg 16:1, January 1979

Malt RA: Portasystemic venous shunts, two parts. N Engl J Med 295: 24, 80, 1976

Mcdermott WV Jr: Surgery of the Liver and Portal Circulation. Philadelphia, Lea & Febiger, 1974

Popper H (ed): Symposium on cirrhosis. Clin Gastroenterol 4:225, 1975

Resnick RH: Portal hypertension. Med Clin North Am 59:945, 1975

QUESTIONS

DIRECTIONS: Each of the questions or incomplete statements below is followed by five suggested answers or completions. Select the *one* that is *best* in each case.

A 45-year-old alcoholic male presents hypotensive with massive upper gastrointestinal bleeding.

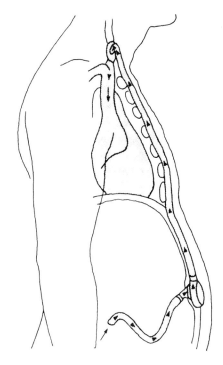

Figure 12-3 LeVeen continuous peritoneojugular shunt.

1. The most likely physical finding if this bleeding results from esophageal varices is:
   A. Ascites
   B. Pancreatic pseudocyst
   C. Palpable thrill over umbilical vein
   D. Splenomegaly
   E. Jaundice
2. After institution of resuscitative measures, the first diagnostic study that should be undertaken is:
   A. Upper gastrointestinal series
   B. Celiac angiography
   C. Measurement of portal pressure by splenic pulp manometry
   D. Measurement of portal pressure by hepatic wedge pressure
   E. Esophagogastroscopy
3. The least likely of the following to be a complication of use of the Sengstaken-Blakemore tube is:
   A. Laceration of varices
   B. Esophageal rupture
   C. Aspiration pneumonia
   D. Asphyxia
   E. Esophageal and gastric ulceration
4. If bleeding continues despite all medical measures, the most *rapid* surgical measure for control of variceal hemorrhage would be:
   A. End-to-side portacaval shunt

   B. Side-to-side portacaval shunt
   C. Warren shunt
   D. Splenectomy
   E. Variceal ligation
5. As the above procedure will result in a high incidence of recurrent bleeding,
   a possible alternative technique for rapid control of variceal hemorrhage
   would be:
   A. Subcardiac portoazygous disconnection
   B. Mesocaval shunt
   C. Distal splenorenal shunt
   D. Portacaval shunt with arterialization
   E. Central splenorenal shunt
6. The Budd-Chiari syndrome (postsinusoidal) is best treated with:
   A. End-to-side portacaval shunt
   B. Side-to-side portacaval shunt
   C. Warren shunt
   D. Splenectomy
   E. Variceal ligation
7. Which of the following findings is consistent with a Child's "C"
   classification?
   A. Albumin = 2.5 g percent
   B. Bilirubin = 2.5 mg percent
   C. Mild ascites
   D. Minimal encephalopathy
   E. All of these
8. Which of the following is physiologically different from the others?
   A. Mesocaval shunt
   B. Mesorenal shunt
   C. Side-to-side portacaval shunt
   D. Central splenorenal shunt
   E. Distal splenorenal shunt
9. The lowest incidence of encephalopathy will follow the:
   A. End-to-side portacaval shunt
   B. Side-to-side portacaval shunt
   C. Central splenorenal shunt
   D. Distal splenorenal shunt
   E. Mesocaval H-graft
10. "Arterialization" is best used in conjunction with:
    A. End-to-side portacaval shunt
    B. Side-to-side portacaval shunt
    C. Portoazygous disconnection
    D. Central splenorenal shunt
    E. Distal splenorenal shunt
11. The most important etiologic factor in cirrhotic portal hypertension is:
    A. Reduction in volume of hepatic microcirculation
    B. Hepatic cell necrosis
    C. Regenerating nodule formation
    D. Fibrous septa
    E. Intrahepatic shunting

12. The most satisfactory surgical approach to ascites in a patient with normal renal function is:
    A. Side-to-side portacaval shunt
    B. End-to-side portacaval shunt
    C. Mesocaval shunt
    D. Peritoneojugular shunt
    E. Thoracic duct drainage

ANSWERS

1. **D** The most common physical sign of cirrhosis appears to be splenomegaly, occurring in 80 to 90 percent of patients.
2. **E** Esophagogastroscopy is most likely to rapidly reveal the source of massive upper gastrointestinal hemorrhage. A large Ewald tube may be used to copiously irrigate blood and clots from the stomach.
3. **A** If the patient complains of substernal chest pain during inflation of the gastric balloon, it may be in the esophagus and should be immediately deflated. Another lumen or another tube should be placed above the Sengstaken tube within the esophagus to aspirate secretions. A heavy scissors should be kept at the bedside at all times to allow rapid transection and removal of the tube if it slips so that the inflated balloon causes respiratory obstruction.
4. **E** Variceal ligation provides a rapid method of stopping hemorrhage, but its incidence of rebleeding is high.
5. **B** Of the shunts, the mesocaval H-graft is the most rapid. Portoazygous disconnection has a high incidence of rebleeding.
6. **B** The side-to-side portacaval shunt allows decompression of the intrahepatic venous system through backflow in the portal vein and thus is valuable in the treatment of hepatic vein obstruction (Budd-Chiari) syndrome.
7. **A**
8. **E** The distal splenorenal shunt does not totally divert portal flow from the liver and, hence, results in lower incidence of encephalopathy. The others are *functional* side-to-side portacaval shunts.
9. **D**
10. **A** "Arterialization" is performed by a jump graft from the gastroepiploic artery to the hepatic stump of the portal vein. Its function is to increase hepatic perfusion and hence prevent encephalopathy.
11. **C** There are a number of pathologies resulting in the portal hypertension of cirrhosis, but it appears that regenerating nodule formations with their resultant pressure is most important in microcirculatory obstruction.
12. **D** By far.

13. Pancreas

ANATOMY

1. Parts: head, body, tail, uncinate process
2. Ducts (See Fig. 13-1)
   a. Wirsung—enters duodenum with common bile duct
   b. Santorini—2.5 cm proximal to ampulla of Vater
3. Blood supply (See Fig. 13-2)
   a. Celiac →
      i. Splenic → dorsal pancreatic, pancreatica magna, caudal pancreatic
      ii. Hepatic → gastroduodenal → pancreaticoduodenal
   b. Superior mesenteric artery

PHYSIOLOGY

1. Exocrine
   a. Secretin-stimulated centroacinar and intercalated duct cells: 1-2 liters per day of a clear alkaline solution containing sodium, potassium, water, bicarbonate, chloride
   b. Pancreozymin-stimulated acinar cells
      i. Lipase and amylase secreted in active form
      ii. Proteolytic enzymes activated by enterokinase in duodenum
      iii. Phospholipase A activated by trypsin in duodenum
      iv. Ribonuclease
   c. Prevention of autodigestion
      i. Zymogen granule storage
      ii. Inactive form of enzymes secreted
      iii. Inhibitors of proteolytic enzymes in pancreas
2. Endocrine
   a. Insulin (51 amino acid polypeptide)
   b. Glucagon

ETIOLOGY

1. Biliary (40 percent), *mechanism*
   a. Transient obstruction of ampulla of Vater and pancreatic duct by gallstone
   b. In most cases, choledocholithiasis is *not* found, but gallstone may be found in feces

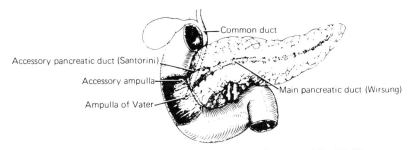

Figure 13-1   Anatomy of the pancreatic ducts. Courtesy of Dr. W. Silen.

2. Alcoholic (40 percent)—least likely with beer—*mechanism*
   a. Decreases incorporation of P-32 into parenchymal phospholipids
   b. Decreases zymogen synthesis
   c. Ultrastructural changes in acinar cells
   d. Stimulates pancreatic secretion
   e. Spasm of sphincter of Oddi
3. Idiopathic (15 percent)
4. Other causes (5 percent)
   a. Hyperparathyroidism—*mechanism*
      i. Increased calcium in pancreatic juice—calculous precipitation and premature activation of proteases
   b. Hyperlipidemia (especially types I and V)—*diagnosis*
      i. Amylase normal in serum (lipids interfere with assay)
      ii. Urine amylase high
      iii. Look for lactescent serum
   c. Postoperative—*usual causes*
      i. Following gastric or biliary surgery

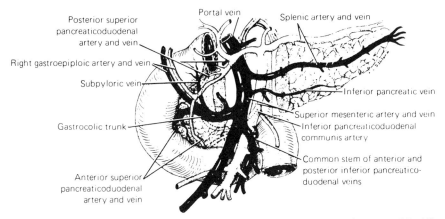

Figure 13-2   Anatomic relationships and blood supply of the pancreas. Courtesy of Dr. W. Silen.

    ii. Especially Bilroth II (not Bilroth I)

    iii. Problem is lack of free drainage from afferent loop

  d. Familial pancreatitis—autosomal dominant

  e. Protein deficiency—mechanism unknown

  f. Steroid therapy

  g. Following ERCP

  h. Pregnancy (usually benign course)

PATHOGENESIS

1. Autodigestion by
   a. Trypsin: activates phospholipase A
   b. Phospholipase A: forms lysolecithin from biliary lecithin → necrotizing pancreatitis
   c. Lipase: fat necrosis
   d. Elastase: digests walls of vessels → hemorrhagic pancreatitis
   e. Blood: when mixed with enzymes heightens inflammatory reaction

MECHANISMS (debated)

1. Obstruction secretion. Induced pancreatic secretion against a *partial* (not complete) pancreatic obstruction
2. Common channel theory: proposed by Claude Bernard in 1856, first case report by Opie in 1901 — problems with this theory
   a. Although functional common channel exists in perhaps 70 percent, few have long enough common channel to allow reflux if ampulla contains stone
   b. Reflux of bile is harmful only if bile contains deconjugated bile salts or is infected
3. Duodenal reflux (unlikely). Reflux of duodenal juice (containing enterokinase) would activate pancreatic enzymes (example Pfeffer loop)
4. Other theories/mechanisms: Trauma, impaired blood supply, autoimmune, lymphatic congestion, activation of kallikrein-kinin system

PATHOPHYSIOLOGY

Ductal hypertension →
Release of enzymes through interlobular spaces →
Alteration of local (then systemic) vasomotor tone →
Increased capillary permeability →
Decreased venous and lymphatic circulation through pancreas →
Impaired portal flow →

Massive fluid loss from pancreas and blood trapped in liver →
Hypovolemia →
Peripheral vasoconstriction (including within pancreas) →
Pancreatic hypoxia →
Pancreatic cell necrosis

COMPLICATIONS

1. Renal failure due to
   a. Hypovolemia and acute tubular necrosis
   b. DIC affecting glomerular tuft
2. Respiratory insufficiency due to
   a. Local factors, such as diaphragmatic irritation or pleural effusion
   b. Serum lecithinase denaturing lecithins of surfactant
3. Endocrine (diabetes)
4. Shock—may be irreversible due to vasoactive substances in hemorrhagic necrotizing pancreatitis
5. Death
   a. 20 to 25 percent in hemorrhagic necrotizing pancreatitis
   b. 1 percent in recurrent acute pancreatitis

CLINICAL FINDINGS

1. Pain (epigastric, back)
2. Vomiting, dehydration
3. Tachycardia, hypotension
4. Abdominal tenderness
5. Abdominal mass (swollen pancreas, pseudocyst, abscess)
6. Pleural effusion (especially left-sided)
7. Bluish discoloration of flank (Grey Turner's sign)
8. Bluish discoloration in periumbilical area (Cullen's sign)

DIAGNOSIS

Bloods
1. Amylase
   a. Serum amylase over 200 IU/ml
      i. In acute pancreatitis, 94 percent of patients have serum amylase over 1875 IU/ml (1000 Somogyi units)
      ii. Nonspecific because elevated also in perforated peptic ulcer, mesenteric infarction, choledocholithiasis, etc.

      iii. Unreliable, not always present in pancreatitis at the time blood sample
         is drawn
  b. Urine amylase over 5000 IU/24 hours
    i. Better in that it gives overall average and hence less time-dependent
      than serum amylase
  c. Amylase clearance/creatinine clearance
    i. Ratio greater than 0.05 in pancreatitis
    ii. Distinguish hyperamylasemia of pancreatitis from other causes
2. Hypocalcemia
3. Hyperbilirubinemia
4. Lipase elevated

X-ray
1. Plain abdominal films
  a. Sentinel loop (dilated bowel adjacent to pancreas)
  b. Colon cutoff sign (colonic spasm in area of pancreas)
  c. Calcification if chronic pancreatis
2. Chest x-ray—pleural effusion
3. UGI series—widened duodenal loop
4. Oral cholecystogram—for cholelithiasis
5. ERCP (endoscopic retrograde cholangiopancreatography)—for evaluation of
  chronic pancreatitis or pseudocyst (See Fig. 13-3)
6. Sonogram—for abscess or pseudocyst
7. Pancreatic scan (selenomethionine)
  a. Nonvisualization → diseased pancreas
  b. Otherwise, not helpful

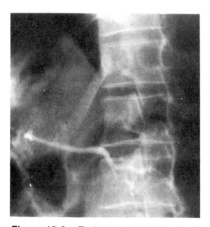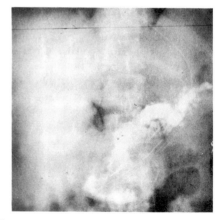

Figure 13-3 Endoscopic retrograde cholangiopancreatography showing normal pancreatic duct (left) and one demonstrating chronic calcific pancreatitis with multiple deformities, strictures, and calcification (right). This patient did well after a longitudinal pancreaticojejunostomy.

MEDICAL THERAPY

Mnemonic → = "PANCREAS" ◄
1. Peritoneal lavage: used in severe refractory cases
2. Analgesics: stay away from morphine and meperidine (spasm of sphincter)
3. Nasogastric tube: helps decrease pancreatic exocrine secretion
4. Calcium: when under 7.5 mg percent, prognosis is poor; if resistant to IV calcium, give parathormone
5. Replacement of fluid and electrolytes: large sequestration of fluid in retroperitoneum; monitor urine output closely
6. Enzyme inhibitor: trasylol (Aprotinin)—inhibits trypsin and kallikrein; efficacy debated
7. Anticholinergics, Antibiotics: not usually used
8. Surgery—usually last resort

OTHER MEDICAL THERAPY (debated)
1. 5-fluorouracil—interferes with protein synthesis within pancreas
2. Fibrinolysin or heparin—to help maintain adequate blood flow to pancreas
3. Glucagon—decreases exocrine secretion, rapidly relieves pain

SURGICAL THERAPY

Indications
1. Diagnosis in doubt
2. No response to medical therapy
3. Abscess or suspected abscess
4. Gastrointestinal hemorrhage (usually a terminal event)
5. Pseudocyst (except some young, small ones that may resolve spontaneously)
6. Intractable pain in chronic pancreatitis
7. Severe malabsorption, steatorrhea, weight loss
8. Refractory obstructive jaundice
9. Pancreatic ascites
10. Suspected carcinoma

Techniques (many)
1. For acute disease
   a. Debridement/drainage—for abscess or necrotizing pancreatitis
   b. Sphincteroplasty, T-tube drainage of CBD, or cholecystostomy—for infected or obstructed biliary tree
2. For chronic disease (See Fig. 13-4)
   a. Longitudinal pancreaticojejunostomy (Puestow-Gillesby procedure)
   b. Caudal pancreaticojejunostomy (DuVal procedure). However, usually there are many points of obstruction (chain of lakes) so that longitudinal would be better
   c. 95 percent distal pancreatectomy

LONGITUDINAL
PANCREATICO-
JEJUNOSTOMY

SPHINCTEROPLASTY

CAUDAL
PANCREATICO-
JEJUNOSTOMY

SUBTOTAL (95%
PANCREATECTOMY)

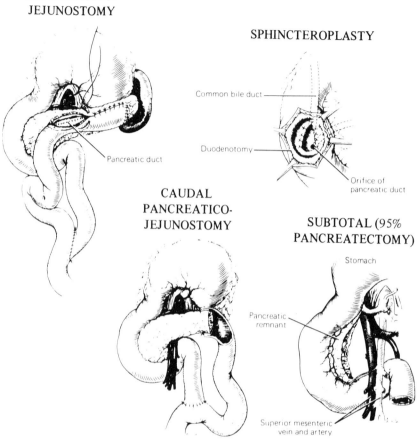

Figure 13-4 Operations currently available for the treatment of chronic pancreatitis. *(From Dunphy JE and Way LW (eds):* Current Surgical diagnosis and Treatment, *3rd Edt. Lange, 1977, p 565, with permission.)*

    d. Whipple procedure (infrequent)

3. For pseudocyst
    a. External drainage—only if wall too thin for internal drainage (before one month this may be the case). Leads to prolonged external fistula
    b. Internal drainage—preferable. Use cystogastrostomy (leak will be acid and dangerous), Roux-en-Y cystojejunostomy (defunctionalized jejunal loop obviates problems with leakage), or cystoduodenostomy

4. For pancreatic ascites
    a. Cause is either leaking pseudocyst, ductal disruption, or occult ductal disruption
    b. Treatment is directed at cause

PANCREATIC NEOPLASMS

INCIDENCE

Rising in the US, M>F

PATHOLOGY

1. Ductal adenocarcinoma—80 percent
2. Cystadenocarcinoma—arises in pseudocyst; good prognosis with radical excision
3. Malignant apudomas

CLINICAL FINDINGS

(in approximate decreasing order of frequency)
1. Head (40 percent)
   a. Pain
   b. Obstructive jaundice
   c. Palpable non-tender gallbladder (Courvoisier's law)—50 percent
   d. Vague deep-seated pain
   e. Pruritis
   f. Hepatomegaly
   g. Back pain
   h. Palpable mass
   i. Sepsis
2. Body (25 percent) and tail (15 percent)
   a. Excruciating paroxysmal pain
   b. Weight loss
   c. Hepatomegaly
   d. Migratory thrombophlebitis (mechanisms unknown)—10 percent
   e. Obstructive jaundice
3. Periampullary (20 percent)
   a. Similar to head, but less weight loss and pain
   b. Jaundice occurs early

DIAGNOSIS

1. Laboratory Findings
   a. Increased alkaline phosphatase and bilirubin—reflect obstructed common bile duct or hepatic metastases
   b. Occult blood in stool

    c. Malignant cytology in duodenal aspirate with secretin stimulation
    d. Oncofetal antigen in serum (new)
 2. X-ray
    a. Often completely negative even in advanced cases!
    b. Hypotonic duodenography—filling defects (reversed 3 sign) or mucosal
       abnormalities
    c. Angiography showing:
       i. "Tumor blush" = hypervascularity within tumor
       ii. Distortion of adjacent vessels
       iii. Regional arterial encasement by tumor mass
    d. ERCP—common bile duct obstruction
    e. CT scan
 3. Tissue Diagnosis by:
       i. Laparotomy with biopsy of mass: fistula is possible complication
       ii. Transduodenal needle biopsy: bleeding or pancreatitis are
           complications
       iii. Fine needle aspiration with cytology
       iv. An extensive inflammatory mass may make diagnosis difficult

THERAPY

 1. Resection for cure is not possible if there is demonstrated involvement of:
    a. Hepatic artery near gastroduodenal artery
    b. Portal or superior mesenteric vein
    c. Superior mesenteric artery
    d. Liver or regional lymph nodes
 2. Whipple operation (pancreaticoduodenectomy) for cancer of head of
    pancreas =
    a. Resection of: antrum, distal common bile duct, gallbladder, duodenum
       and pancreas to mid-body
    b. Truncal vagotomy
    c. Reconstruction by pancreaticojejunostomy, gastrojejunostomy, and
       choledochojejunostomy
    d. Operative mortality—10 to 15 percent
 3. Total Pancreatectomy
    a. Resect as above but include all of pancreas
    b. Reconstruct with choledochojejunostomy and gastrojejunostomy
    c. Rationale for cancer of head of pancreas is that:
       i. 40 percent are multicentric lesions
       ii. Tumor may spread by intraductal and perineural roots within the
           gland
       iii. Eliminates pancreaticojejunostomy which is the major source of
            morbidity
    d. Problems: brittle diabetes mellitus, and exocrine insufficiency
 4. Palliative procedures: cholecystojejunostomy; choledochojejunostomy;
    gastrojejunostomy; radiotherapy; combined chemotherapy

COMPLICATIONS

1. Direct spread with obstruction of:
   a. Duodenum
   b. Common bile duct
   c. Splenic vein = splenomegaly and segmental portal hypertension
   d. Hepatic vein = Budd-Chiari syndrome
2. Lymphatic spread
3. Hepatic and lung metastases
4. Peritoneal seeding and ascites
5. Death: 5-year *survival* is 2.5 percent (30 percent if periampullary)

SELECTED BIBLIOGRAPHY

Cooperman A, Hoerr SD: Surgery of the Pancreas. St Louis, Mosby, 1977
Moosa AR (ed): Tumors of the Pancreas. Baltimore, Williams & Wilkens, 1980

QUESTIONS

1. A 40-year-old male patient who has been drinking one pint of hard liquor daily for the past 20 years presents with severe epigastric pain radiating to the back and associated with nausea and vomiting. He has no previous hospital admissions. The radiologic study most likely to be of value during the acute phase of this disease is:
   A. Pancreatic scan
   B. Oral cholecystogram
   C. Plain film of the abdomen
   D. Endoscopic retrograde cholangiopancreatography
   E. Liver scan
2. The enzyme thought to be most important in the pathogenesis of necrotizing pancreatitis is:
   A. Phospholipase A
   B. Elastase
   C. Trypsin
   D. Lipase
   E. Amylase
3. Current theory concerning the etiology of the respiratory insufficiency of pancreatitis implicates:
   A. Massive pleural effusion
   B. Necrosis of lung parenchyma due to circulating amylase
   C. Chemical pneumonia
   D. Bronchospasm
   E. Denatured surfactant
4. Of the following, the procedure most likely to be complicated by postoperative acute pancreatitis is:
   A. Gastrectomy and Bilroth I reconstruction

    B. Gastrectomy and Bilroth II reconstruction
    C. Vagotomy and pyloroplasty
    D. Parietal cell vagotomy
    E. Cholecystectomy

5. A 45-year-old alcoholic male with symptomatic severe calcific pancreatitis involving multiple segments of the pancreatic duct is best treated operatively with a:
    A. DuVal procedure (caudal pancreaticojejunostomy)
    B. Total pancreatectomy
    C. Whipple procedure
    D. Splanchnicectomy
    E. Longitudinal pancreaticojejunostomy

6. A 50-year-old male with alcoholic pancreatitis is explored electively for treatment of a pseudocyst of the tail of the pancreas. After opening the cyst during the performance of a cystojejunostomy, a suspicious-appearing lesion is noted on the cyst lining. Biopsy reveals cystadenocarcinoma. No suspicious lymph nodes are seen. The appropriate therapy at this point is:
    A. External drainage
    B. Roux-en-Y cystojejunostomy
    C. Radical excision
    D. Biopsy alone
    E. Chemotherapeutic infusion via hepatic artery cannulation

7. Thrombophlebitis migrans is associated most commonly with which one of the following?
    A. Insulinoma
    B. WDHA syndrome
    C. Cancer of the head of the pancreas
    D. Cancer of the body of the pancreas
    E. Pancreatico pseudocyst

DIRECTIONS: For each of the questions or incomplete statements below, *one* or *more* of the answers or completions given is correct. Select:

    A if only *1, 2, and 3* are correct
    B if only *1 and 3* are correct
    C if only *2 and 4* are correct
    D if only *4* is correct
    E if all are correct

---

8. Arteriographic signs of pancreatic cancer include:
    1. Regional arterial encasement
    2. "Tumor stain"
    3. Adjacent arterial displacement
    4. Occlusion of the celiac axis

9. The reasons for the recommendation of some surgeons of total pancreatectomy over the Whipple procedure in cancer of the head of the pancreas include:
    1. Multicentricity in 40 percent
    2. Perineural spread

3. Intraductal spread
4. Elimination of pancreaticojejunostomy

DIRECTIONS: Group of items below consists of five lettered headings followed by a list of numbered phrases. For *each* numbered phrase, select the *one* lettered heading that is most closely associated with it. Each lettered heading or lettered component may be selected once, more than once, or not at all.

A Cancer of the body of the pancreas
B Cancer of the tail of the pancreas
C Malignant Apudoma
D Cystoadenocarcinoma
E Periampulary cancer

---

10. Early jaundice
11. Arises in pseudocyst
12. Streptozotocin may be of therapeutic value

ANSWERS

1. **C** An abdominal flat plate may show the sentinel loop or the colon cutoff sign, or reveal an abscess or pseudocyst. Even radiopaque pancreatic or biliary calculi may show up. Pancreatic scan is meaningful only in the case of complete nonvisualization. OCG and ERCP are not performed during the acute attack.

2. **A** Phospholipase A is the enzyme thought at this time to be most culpable in the pathogenesis of acute pancreatitis. After activation by trypsin, it converts biliary lecithin to lysolecithin, which leads to necrotizing pancreatitis.

3. **E** While local factors such as pleural effusion or inflammation of the diaphragm may contribute to the respiratory problems of pancreatitis, severe respiratory distress syndrome in pancreatitis is thought to result from denaturing of pulmonary surfactant by serum lecithinase.

4. **B** Bilroth II reconstructions are apt to result in pancreatitis in the event of afferent loop obstruction.

5. **E** Calcific pancreatitis in multiple areas of the duct ("chain of lakes") is best treated by longitudinal pancreaticojejunostomy (Puestow-Gillesby procedure).

6. **C** Survival after radical excision of a cystadenocarcinoma is better than that after ductal adenocarcinoma of the pancreas.

7. **D** Thrombophlebitis migrans occurs in approximately 10% of patients with cancer of the body or tail of the pancreas. The etiology is unknown.

8. **A**

9. **E**

10. **E**

11. **D**

12. **C**

14. Spleen and Lymphoproliferative Diseases

ANATOMY

1. Weight
   a. 100 to 150 g, decreasing slightly with age
2. Suspensory ligaments
   a. Splenorenal
      i. Contains splenic pedicle at medial edge
   b. Phrenosplenic
   c. Gastrosplenic
      i. From embryologic dorsal mesogastrium
      ii. Where primordial lobulations may persist unfused (accessory spleens)
      iii. Contains short gastric vessels that may be injured during gastric surgery
   d. Phrenocolic
   e. Splenocolic
3. Divided by connective tissue trabeculae
   a. Trabecular arteries →
   b. White pulp (lymphoid follicles with reticular network containing lymphocytes, plasma cells, and macrophages) →
   c. Marginal zone (sequestration of foreign bodies and abnormal cells) →
   d. Red pulp (splenic cords and sinuses) →
   e. Venous drainage: *overall,* acts as a specialized capillary bed between splenic artery and portal venous system.

PHYSIOLOGY

1. Cell entrapment
   a. Each cell passes through spleen about 1000 times daily
   b. Slitlike openings between cords and sinuses trap abnormally shaped cells
   c. "Conditioning" by travel through areas that are hypoxic, acidotic, and glucose-deprived makes weakened cells more likely to be trapped on next passage
2. Hematopoiesis
   a. Extramedullary hematopoiesis occurs in the fetus and in some disease states in adults

b. Monocytes, lymphocytes, and plasma cells in the adult
3. Immune function
   a. Intimate contact of slow-moving plasma with macrophages lining cords and sinuses provides opportunity for immune recognition of antigens
   b. Increased incidence of severe infection after splenectomy especially in infants under 2 years old

DIAGNOSIS

1. Physical examination—splenomegaly detected by:
   a. Palpation
   b. Percussion of dullness at 9th intercostal space in left anterior axillary line
2. Bloods
   a. Hemogram
   b. Red cell survival (using Cr-51 labeled red cells)
3. X-ray
   a. Mediad and caudad displacement of stomach bubble
   b. Posterior and caudad displacement of splenic flexure
4. Scan
   a. Cr-51 labeled autogenous red cells
   b. Radioactive mercury

Disease States Which Sometimes Benefit from Splenectomy

Condition	Findings	Etiology	Therapy
Primary hypersplenism	Pancytopenia Splenomegaly Active marrow	Unknown	Corticosteroids SPLENECTOMY
Secondary hypersplenism	Pancytopenia Splenomegaly Active marrow	Exaggerated normal function of spleen due to intrinsic blood cell defects, cell destruction, or splenomegaly	(1) Treat underlying cause (2) Corticosteroids (3) SPLENECTOMY, for a. Major hemolysis b. WBC under 1000 with infection c. Purpura or hemorrhage due to thrombocytopenia d. Symptomatic massive splenomegaly

(continued)

Condition	Findings	Etiology	Therapy
Hereditary spherocytosis (commonest congenital hemolytic anemia)	Splenomegaly Anemia Jaundice Increased osmotic fragility of RBCs Spherocytes (nonspecific) Hypoplastic crises (rare) Pigment gallstones (85% of adults) Chronic leg ulcers (rare)	Increased sodium and water permeability of RBC membrane — rigid, small, round cells recognized as abnormal by spleen	SPLENECTOMY Look for accessory spleens, inspect gallbladder (prognosis excellent) In children, delay until over five if possible
Hereditary eliptocytosis (ovalocytosis)	Usually asymptomatic Sometimes anemia, jaundice, splenomegaly	Abnormal permeability of RBC membrane	SPLENECTOMY if symptomatic
Acquired hemolytic anemia	Anemia, fever, jaundice, reticulocytosis, erythroid hyperplasia of marrow, decreased haptoglobin, (+) direct Coombs' Gallstones (25%) Splenomegaly (50%) Renal tubular necrosis (rare)	Immunologic alteration of RBCs due to chemicals, bacteria, drugs (penicillin, quinidine, methyldopa)	(1) Stop drug (2) Corticosteroids (3) Blood transfusions (4) SPLENECTOMY for warm (IgG) antibodies
Thalassemia major (Cooley's anemia)	Autosomal dominant Anemia Jaundice Hepatospleno- megaly Retarded body growth Large head Fetal Hgb Gallstones (25%)	Abnormal Hgb → target cells	SPLENECTOMY in some cases
Idiopathic throm- bocytopenic purpura (ITP)	Thrombocytopenia (under 100,000) with normal megakaryocytes Ecchymoses	Circulating antiplatelet factor which is: (1) idiopathic, or (2) secondary to	(1) Mild symptoms → avoid trauma (2) Moderate or severe symptoms → a. Prednisone 40

Condition	Findings	Etiology	Therapy
	Petechiae Bleeding gums Vaginal, GI, GU bleeding CNS bleeding (3%) Chronic form with insidious onset Diagnosis made by exclusion splenomegaly (very rare)	lymphoproli- ferative disorders, drugs, toxins, bacterial or viral infection, systemic lupus	mg daily until plat ct normal, b. SPLENECTOMY for no response to steroid, relapses; disease lasting more than one year; intracranial bleeding Succeeds in 70%, if failure use c. Azathioprine or vincristine
Thrombotic cytopenic purpura (TTP)	Fever Thrombocytopenia Purpura Hemolytic anemia Neurologic mani- festations Renal failure Hepatospleno- megaly (35%) Gingival biopsy diagnostic Death (90%)	Autoimmune (?)	Heparin, dextran, steroids, SPLENECTOMY (? No real cure)
Agnogenic myeloid metaplasia	Massive spleno- megaly (100%) Hepatomegaly (75%) Leukoerythro- blastic blood reaction Anemia Abdominal fullness, pain	Idiopathic	(1) Transfusion (2) Androgenic steroids (3) Antimetabolites (4) Radiotherapy (5) SPLENECTOMY for major hemolysis unresponsive to medical therapy; dangerous thrombo- cytopenia; portal hypertension with variceal bleed; symptomatic massive splenomegaly Associated with 13% mortality
Splenic artery aneurysm	Usu. asymptomatic Calcification on	(1) Congenital (2) Atherosclerosis	SPLENECTOMY except in

(continued)

Condition	Findings	Etiology	Therapy
	abdominal films Occas. pain, nausea, vomiting Rarely, rupture (especially in pregnancy)	(3) Inflammatory process (e.g., pancreatitis)	asymptomatic patients over 60 years old
Neoplasms	Calcification on x-ray Splenomegaly Eosinophilia Palpable mass	Echinococcal cyst Dermoid, epidermoid, endothelial or pseudocyst Lymphoma Sarcoma Hemangioma Hamartoma Metastasis	SPLENECTOMY, except for metastasis
Abscess	Sepsis Splenomegaly Abdominal pain Splenic scan or arteriogram Gas in spleen on plain x-ray	(1) Hematogenous seeding (2) Direct spread (3) Trauma with hematoma	SPLENECTOMY Splenotomy with drainage for large abscess in some cases
Ectopic spleen	Mass Acute torsion may occur	Long pedicle	SPLENECTOMY
Rupture	Shock Abdominal pain Pain referred to (L) shoulder or neck (Kehr's sign) Nausea, vomiting Tenderness over (L) 9, 10 ribs Paracentesis	(1) Antecedent trauma (2) Sometimes spontaneous (3) Operative trauma (4) Delayed rupture (5% of blunt injuries to spleen)	SPLENECTOMY (Increasing concern about immunologic function of spleen has led to some attempts at splenic repair for trauma)

HODGKIN'S DISEASE

1. Classification (Ann Arbor system)
   a. Stage I: single lymph node region (I); single extralymphatic organ or site (Ie)
   b. Stage II: two or more node regions on same side of diaphragm (II); extralymphatic organ or side *and* one or more lymph node regions on same side of diaphragm (IIe)
   c. Stage III: node regions on both sides of diaphragm (III); + splenic involvement (IIIs); + localized extralymphatic organ or site (IIIe); + both (IIIse)

   d. Stage IV: diffuse or disseminated involvement of one or more extralymphatic organs or sites

   e. Fever, night sweats, and/or unexplained weight loss of more than 10 percent of body weight in the six months prior to admission

     a. If present, suffix B to stage number

     b. If absent, suffix A to stage number

2. Clinical presentation

   a. Painless lymphadenopathy- cervical most common- 80 percent

   b. Fever (classical Pel-Ebstein fever curve is uncommon)

   c. Malaise, weight loss

   d. Tracheal compression

   e. Pruritis

   f. Pain in involved lymph nodes occurring after alcohol intake lasting until metabolism of the ethanol—mechanism unknown

3. Methods for clinical staging (See Fig. 14-1)

"BLOOD, BONES, LIVER SCAN;
CHEST, NODES, LYMPHANGIOGRAM" ◄

   a. BLOOD: hematologic tests

   b. BONES: bone marrow aspiration and biopsy; bone survery, scan

   c. LIVER SCAN: Tc-99 scan, CT scan; also liver function tests; if hepatic involvement strongly suspected, percutaneous or laparoscopic liver biopsy is undertaken

   d. CHEST: x-ray to detect lung or mediastinal involvement; may require tomography for confirmation

   e. NODES: examine all accessible lymph nodes including *Waldeyer's ring;* biopsy for confirmation of diagnosis

   f. LYMPHANGIOGRAM: bipedal lymphangiogram to detect paraaortic node involvement; however, only about 80 percent accurate

4. Indications for staging laparotomy (required in most cases)

   a. When result of laparotomy may change therapy

   b. Symptomatic splenomegaly

5. Contraindications for staging laparotomy

   a. Stage IV already documented

   b. When surgery contraindicated for medical reasons

   c. Lymphocytic predominant histology and negative lymphangiogram

   d. Mediastinal lymphadenopathy without cervical or supraclavicular adenopathy

6. Performance of staging laparotomy

   a. SPLENECTOMY

   b. Liver biopsies

   c. Numerous lymph node biopsies

   d. Mark biopsy sites with metal clips

   e. Thorough abdominal exploration

   f. Retrouterine oophoropexy

   g. Iliac crest wedge bone biopsy

7. Change of staging with laparotomy

   a. Usually to more advanced stage: at laparotomy, spleen: positive → negative 65 percent; negative → positive 30 percent

120

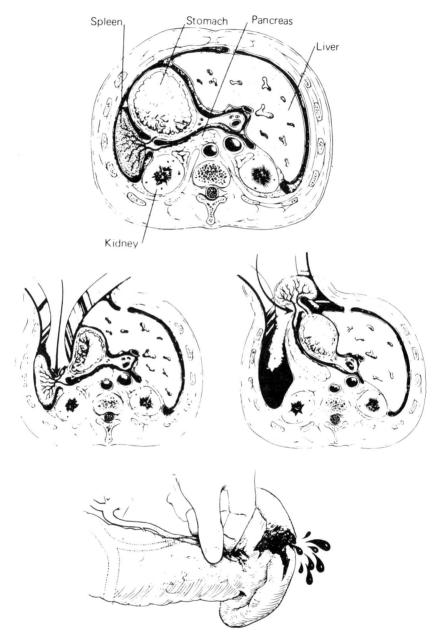

Figure 14-1 Normal anatomic relationships of the spleen (top), technique for routine splenectomy (middle), and method for rapid control of hemorrhage due to splenic laceration by grasping the tail of the pancreas within the lesser sac (bottom). *(From Dunphy FE and Way LW (eds):* Current Surgical Diagnosis and Treatment, *3rd Edt. Lange, 1977, pp 571 and 583, and Artz CP and Hardy JD:* Management of Surgical Complications, *3rd Edt. W.B. Saunders Co., 1975, p 564, with permission.)*

Prognosis
1. Continues to improve
2. At present five-year survival is over 80 percent except in stage IV

NON-HODGKIN'S LYMPHOMAS

Differ from Hodgkin's disease in the following
1. Commonly in the very young and very old
2. Not usually associated with fever or pruritis, but often causes general deterioration of the patient
3. Rarely involves sternal nodes but often involves bilateral upper cervical, jugular, and spinal chains, and often leads to rather voluminous lymphadenopathy
4. May primarily involve the gastrointestinal tract or upper airway
5. Shows an immediate response to irradiation
7. Diagnostic work-up: Similar to that of Hodgkin's lymphoma, but intensive, non-invasive staging will elevate most patients to Stage III or IV. Systemic therapy is more commonly used in the treatment of Stage III. These two factors limit laparotomy to < 20 percent
8. Treatment: Stages I and II → radiotherapy, Stages III and IV → chemotherapy
9. Prognosis: Poorer than in Hodgkin's disease—five-year survival in localized disease is 50 percent and much less for extensive disease. Reticulum cell sarcoma has a grave prognosis

TECHNIQUES OF SPLENECTOMY (See Fig. 14-2)

1. Mobilize, then tie splenic artery by posterior dissection in hilum, or
2. Tie splenic artery first within lesser sac to allow autotransfusion before delivering spleen, and to lessen size of enlarged spleen
3. Drainage is debated, but indicated at least in myeloid metaplasia because massive splenomegaly → large potential space

COMPLICATIONS OF SPLENECTOMY

1. Hematologic
   a. Red cells may have Howell-Jolly bodies or Heinz bodies or be siderocytes, but count and indices should not change
   b. Platelet count may rise to 400,000 to 500,000 for one year
      i. No therapy is required
      ii. Aspirin may be of benefit for count over 1,000,000
   c. Antibody production temporarily decreased
      i. IgM levels are down for over three years
      ii. In children, may be associated with severe or fatal sepsis usually due to pneumococcus, meningococcus, or Hemophilus influenza
   d. Leukocytosis, especially lymphocytosis

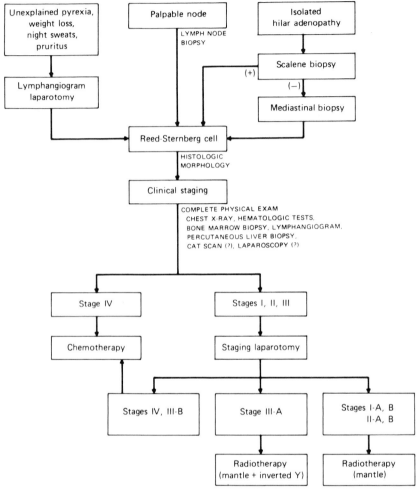

Figure 14-2 Hodgkin's Disease: Diagnostic and treatment pathways. The rationale in treatment is that nodal disease is curable by sterilizing doses of radiation, while diffuse disease (Stage IV) or occult disease (B stages) require systemic chemotherapy.

2. Operative complications
    a. Pancreatitis
    b. Left lower lobe atelectasis
    c. Subphrenic hematoma → abscess
    d. Hemorrhage
    e. Thromboembolism
    f. Gastric perforation
3. Other
    a. Failure of splenectomy to relieve hematologic disorder. Usually due to missed accessory spleen

SELECTED BIBLIOGRAPHY

Dameshek HL, et al.: Hematologic indications for splenectomy. Surg Clin North Am 55:253, 1975
Schwartz SI, et al.: Splenectomy for hematologic disorders. Curr Probl Surg May 1971
Stillman RM: The role of surgery in lymphoproliferative disease. In Alfonso AE, Gardner B: Practice of Cancer Surgery. New York, Appleton-Century-Crofts, 1982, p 281

QUESTIONS

DIRECTIONS: Each of the questions or incomplete statements below is followed by five suggested answers or completions. Select the *one* that is *best* in each case.

1. Splenectomy is least likely to benefit a patient with:
   A. Agnogenic myeloid metaplasia
   B. Hereditary spherocytosis
   C. Splenic artery aneurysm
   D. Thrombotic thrombocytopenic purpura
   E. Primary hypersplenism
2. A 16-year-old female with pigment gallstones most likely has:
   A. Hereditary spherocytosis
   B. Sickle cell anemia
   C. Elliptocytosis
   D. Acquired hemolytic anemia
   E. Thalassemia major
3. A five-year-old child developing serious sepsis following splenectomy most likely is infected with:
   A. Meningococcus
   B. Hemophilus influenza
   C. A virus
   D. *E. coli*
   E. Pneumococcus

DIRECTIONS: For each of the questions or incomplete statements below, *one* or *more* of the answers or completions given is correct. Select:
   A if only 1, 2, *and* 3 are correct
   B if only 1 *and* 3 are correct
   C if only 2 *and* 4 are correct
   D if only 4 is correct
   E if all are correct

4. Expected hematologic parameters after splenectomy performed for hereditary spherocytosis include:
   1. Continued spherocytosis
   2. Persistent osmotic fragility

   3. Normal tagged red cell survival
   4. Persistent anemia
 5. True of idiopathic thrombocytopenic purpura:
   1. Often a self-limiting process
   2. Hemolytic anemia usually present
   3. Emergency splenectomy sometimes indicated
   4. Bone marrow failure is a prominent factor
 6. Staging laparotomy in adult Hodgkin's disease:
   1. Rarely changes clinical staging
   2. Does not include splenectomy if spleen is grossly normal
   3. Greatly increases risk of fatal sepsis
   4. Cannot differentiate stage IA from stage IIA
 7. True of congenital hemolytic anemia:
   1. Increased osmotic fragility of erythrocytes
   2. Positive direct Coombs' test
   3. Splenomegaly
   4. Splenectomy contraindicated in all cases
 8. True of acquired hemolytic anemia:
   1. Positive direct Coombs' test
   2. Increased osmotic fragility of erythrocytes
   3. Splenomegaly
   4. Splenectomy contraindicated in all cases
 9. A 26-year-old female having her first episode of severe vaginal bleeding is
    found to have ITP with a platelet count of 50,000. Initial therapy should
    include:
   1. Splenectomy
   2. Blood transfusion
   3. Azathioprine
   4. Corticosteroid therapy
10. Indications for splenectomy in ITP include:
   1. First episode unresponsive to steroid therapy
   2. Multiple episodes, each responsive to steroid therapy
   3. Symptomatic thrombocytopenia lasting over one year
   4. Intracranial bleeding

ANSWERS

 1. **D** TTP is a fatal disease in which various therapies including splenectomy
           have been attempted with little success.
 2. **A** Hereditary spherocytosis leads to pigment gallstones in 85 percent of
           adult cases. Children with pigment stones most likely have
           spherocytosis. Treatment is splenectomy and cholecystectomy.
 3. **E**
 4. **A** The anemia will resolve as a result of normal red cell life span after
           splenectomy. Spherocytosis and osmotic fragility, a result of abnormal
           red cell membrane permeability, persist.

5. **B** Emergency splenectomy is indicated in ITP for thrombocytopenia with life-threatening hemorrhage. Especially in children, it is often a self-limiting process (which may result from a viral infection). Bone marrow failure is not a problem (normal megakaryocytes).
6. **D** Stage I and II both are disease above the diaphragm and therefore cannot be differentiated. This procedure changes clinical staging in about one-third of cases, usually to a higher stage. Includes splenectomy in all cases (error in gross assessment of disease is substantial).
7. **B** Congenital spherocytosis is the most common type of congenital hemolytic anemia.
8. **B**
9. **C** Blood transfusion for massive bleeding and prednisone therapy.
10. **E** All are indications for splenectomy in ITP.

15. Hernia

ANATOMY

1. Layers of abdominal wall in inguinal area
   a. Scarpa's fascia: thickest in inguinal area
   b. External oblique muscle/aponeurosis
      i. From lower eight ribs to inguinal ligament
   ▶ ii. "Runs in the direction you put your hands in your pockets"
   c. Internal oblique muscle: from lateral half of inguinal ligament to pubic tubercle
   d. Transversalis muscle/fascia
      i. Thickest portion = iliopubic tract
      ii. Internal ring is formed by embryonic herniation of processus vaginalis through this layer
   e. Conjoined tendon (falx inguinalis) = tendinous thickened portion of internal oblique + transversalis
2. Important structures in inguinal area
   a. External ring
      i. Opening in external oblique aponeurosis
      ii. Carries ilioinguinal nerve + spermatic cord or round ligament
   b. Lacunar (Gimbernat) ligament: triangular reflection of lower inguinal ligament from pubic tubercle along iliopectineal line
   c. Cooper's ligament: strong fibrous band along iliopectineal line on superior pubic ramus
   d. Internal ring
      i. Bordered superiorly by internal oblique
      ii. Inferiorly and medially by inferior epigastric vessels
   e. Hesselbach's triangle: bordered by inguinal ligament, inferior epigastric vessels, conjoined tendon
   f. Femoral triangle: bordered by inguinal ligament, sartorius muscle, pectineus and adductor magnus muscles

CLASSIFICATION

1. General
   a. Reducible
   b. Incarcerated = irreducible
   c. Strangulated = interference with blood supply to incarcerated organ
   d. Sliding = wall of viscus forms wall of sac, more frequent on left side, cecum or sigmoid usually (See Fig. 15-1)
      i. Intrasaccular = mesentery to sac

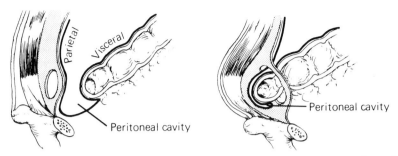

Figure 15-1 Formation of sliding right indirect inguinal hernia. *(From Dunphy JE and Way LW (eds):* Current Surgical Diagnosis and Treatment, *3rd Edt. Lange, 1977, p 682, with permission.)*

  ii. Parasaccular (intramural) = organ forms portion of sac wall—most common type 95 percent
  iii. Extrasaccular (usually bladder) = extraperitoneal, easily separated
  e. Richter's = incarceration of only a portion of bowel wall. Danger is perforation without intestinal obstruction
2. Specific
  a. Indirect inguinal = sac anteromedial to cord through internal ring
  b. Direct inguinal = through Hesselbach's triangle
  c. Femoral = through femoral canal beneath inguinal ligament
  d. Pantaloon = combination direct/indirect inguinal
  e. Umbilical
  f. Incisional
  g. Spigelian = through linea semilunaris
  h. Littre's = sac contains Meckel's diverticulum
  i. Obturator = through obturator canal
  j. Sciatic = through foramen of greater sciatic nerve
  k. Lumbar = usually in Petit's triangle
  l. Interparietal = between layers of abdominal wall
  m. Perineal = through perineum

INCIDENCE

1. Most common is *indirect inguinal* in either male or female. However, femoral hernias comprise 33 percent of groin hernias in females, but only 2 percent in males
2. Inguinal hernias more commonly on right than left (related to previous appendectomy?)

ETIOLOGY

1. Indirect inguinal: congenitally present sac (processus vaginalis)
2. Direct inguinal: acquired weakness in floor of Hesselbach's triangle
3. Femoral: congenitally narrow attachment of posterior inguinal wall to Cooper's ligament

ASSOCIATED FACTORS

1. Obesity, age, chronic disease
2. Abdominal pressure increase
   a. Chronic constipation
   b. Chronic cough or sneeze
   c. Straining on urination (prostatism)
   d. Ascites
   e. Pregnancy
3. Intraabdominal pathology: colon carcinoma (very rare)—*routine* proctoscopy debated, routine barium enema not indicated

DIAGNOSIS

1. History of recurrent mass, pain
2. Palpable mass

TREATMENT OF INGUINAL/FEMORAL HERNIA

Key is to Close Defect in Transversalis Fascia
1. High ligation of sac alone is sufficient for indirect hernia in children
2. Bassini
   a. Conjoined tendon and transversalis fascia sutured to shelving border of inguinal ligament
3. McVay
   a. Relaxing incision in anterior rectus shealth
   b. Suture conjoined tendon to Cooper's ligament medially
   c. Suture iliopubic tract to inguinal ligament laterally to avoid compression of femoral vein
   d. Considered a stronger and more anatomic repair (See Fig 15-2)
4. Shouldice
   a. Transversalis fascia divided longitudinally
   b. Imbricated in two layers to inguinal ligament
   c. Conjoined tendon to external oblique fascia in double layer
5. Properitoneal technique
   a. Open rectus shealth and transversalis fascia 4 cm above inguinal ligament
   b. Exposes inguinal canal posteriorly
   c. Useful in recurrent or complicated hernias
   d. Some reports of very high recurrence rates
6. Femoral hernia repair
   a. Reduction may require division of lacunar ligament
   b. Watch for aberrant obturator artery on lateral edge
7. Sliding hernia
   a. Must recognize slider to protect viscus and its blood supply
   b. Bevan technique for partial resection of sac

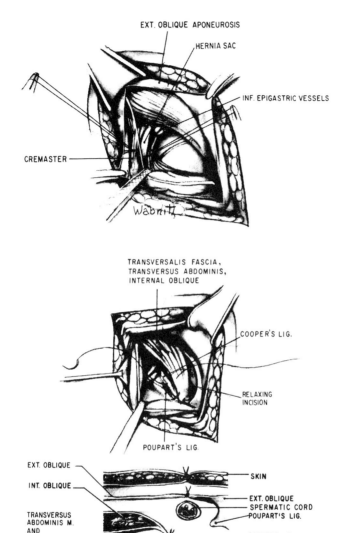

Figure 15-2   Steps in repair of indirect inguinal hernia: high ligation of sac (A), closure of defect in transversalis fascia, by McVay (B).

   c. LaRoque combined abdominal-inguinal approach for reduction of difficult
      sliders
8. Mesh repair
   a. Usually polypropylene (Marlex)
   b. Useful if unable to bring fascia together without tension

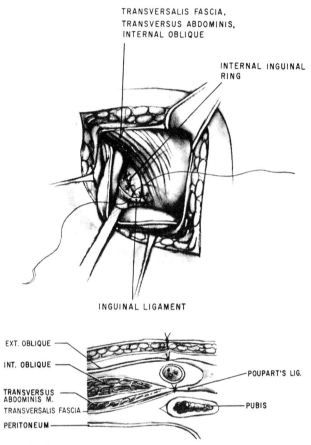

TRANSVERSALIS FASCIA,
TRANSVERSUS ABDOMINIS,
INTERNAL OBLIQUE

INTERNAL INGUINAL
RING

INGUINAL LIGAMENT

EXT. OBLIQUE

INT. OBLIQUE

POUPART'S LIG.

TRANSVERSUS
ABDOMINIS M.
TRANSVERSALIS FASCIA

PUBIS

PERITONEUM

Figure 15-2 (Cont.)   Bassini technique (C). *(From Schwartz SI (ed):* Principles of Surgery, *2nd Edt. McGraw-Hill, 1974, pp 1347 and 1356, with permission.)*

OTHER CONSIDERATIONS

1. Bilateral inguinal hernia: simultaneous repair *only* for small indirect hernias
2. Direct hernia: sac inverted, not excised
3. Resection of spermatic cord in elderly patients:
    a. May be of value in selected recurrent hernias to allow complete obliteration of internal ring, *but*
    b. Results in testicular atrophy, pain, hydrocele
4. Selective nonoperative reduction of incarcerated hernia
    a. Femoral hernia—NEVER!
    b. Other—by Trendelenburg position, sedation
    c. Allows better preoperative preparation
    d. Complication is reduction "en masse" (rare)—i.e., with sac

5. Giant scrotal hernia: use preoperative progressive pneumoperitoneum to avoid postoperative pulmonary and cardiac insufficiency

RECURRENCE

1. Reasons
   a. Failure to recognize associated hernia
   b. Wound infection
   c. Underlying condition causing increased intraabdominal pressure
   d. Error in technique
      i. Excessive tension on suture line (especially due to failure to use relaxing incision in McVay repair)
      ii. Failure to skeletonize cord
      iii. Failure to close internal ring properly
2. Rates
   a. Varies between series (1 to 5 percent)
   b. Most with repair of recurrent hernia
   c. Increases with time

SELECTED BIBLIOGRAPHY

McVay CB: The anatomic basis for inguinal and femoral hernioplasty. SGO 139:931, 1974
Nyhus LM, Condon RE (eds): Hernias, 2nd edt. New York, Lippincott, 1978
Ponka JL: Hernias of the Abdominal Wall. Philadelphia, Saunders, 1980

QUESTIONS

DIRECTIONS: Each of the questions or incomplete statements below is followed by five suggested answers or completions. Select the *one* that is *best* in each case.

A 70-year-old male presents with a long-standing large left scrotal hernia containing sigmoid colon on abdominal x-ray.
1. On exploration, he will most likely be found to have a:
   A. Richter's hernia
   B. Strangulated hernia
   C. Direct hernia
   D. Sliding hernia
   E. Femoral hernia
2. If his medical condition precludes immediate operative repair, the use of a truss may make later herniorraphy difficult due to:
   A. Compromise of colonic blood supply
   B. Dilatation of internal ring

    C. Breakdown of overlying skin
    D. Fibrosis of inguinal canal
    E. Testicular atrophy

3. A 25-year-old male presents with a tender right inguinal hernia, abdominal pain, and a temperature of 101°F. Abdominal x-ray shows multiple differential air/fluid levels. Appropriate initial management is:
    A. Operation
    B. Long-tube intestinal decompression
    C. Nasogastric tube and observation for 24 hours
    D. Barium enema
    E. Sedation and attempted nonoperative reduction

4. The best way to differentiate an infected inguinal lymph node from a strangulated femoral hernia is:
    A. Gallium scan
    B. Sonogram
    C. Barium enema
    D. Response to antibiotics
    E. Operation

5. A 35-year-old multiparous female presents with a reducible groin mass. On exploration she will most likely be found to have a(n):
    A. Femoral hernia
    B. Direct hernia
    C. Indirect hernia
    D. Sliding hernia
    E. Hydrocele

6. Reduction of a femoral hernia by division of Gimbernat's ligament may result in hemorrhage due to laceration of which vessel?
    A. Femoral artery
    B. Inferior epigastric artery
    C. Aberrant obturator artery
    D. Femoral vein
    E. External iliac artery

7. In how many patients having inguinal hernia as their sole complaint will routine barium enema reveal unsuspected colonic carcinoma?
    A. Less than 1:100
    B. 2:100
    C. 5:100
    D. 10:100
    E. More than 10:100

8. Which structure forms a border for both Hesselbach's triangle and the femoral triangle?
    A. Inferior epigastric vessels
    B. Conjoined tendon
    C. Sartorius muscle
    D. Inguinal ligament
    E. None of these

9. Which of the following is *not* a factor resulting in recurrent inguinal hernia?
    A. Failure to use relaxing incision in Cooper's ligament repair
    B. Failure to properly approximate internal ring

C. Failure to recognize associated hernia
D. Use of absorbable suture material
E. Failure to properly approximate external ring

DIRECTIONS: The group of items below consists of five lettered headings, followed by a list of numbered words or phrases. For *each* numbered word or phrase, select the *one* lettered heading or lettered component that is most closely associated with it. Each lettered heading or lettered component may be selected once, more than once, or not at all.

A   Littre's hernia
B   Richter's hernia
C   Petit's triangle hernia
D   Pantaloon hernia
E   Spigelian hernia

---

10. Antimesenteric border of bowel in sac
11. Linea semilunaris defect
12. Lumbar hernia
13. Contains Meckel's diverticulum
14. Combination direct and indirect inguinal hernia

ANSWERS

1. **D** Probably sliding indirect hernia.
2. **D** A truss may result in fibrosis and obliteration of normal anatomy.
3. **A** An incarcerated hernia with abdominal pain and fever suggests a strangulated hernia which requires urgent operative intervention.
4. **E** Any extremely tender inguinal mass should be suspected to be a strangulated femoral hernia and operation should be promptly undertaken. If it turns out to be an infected lymph node, little is lost, while if an incarcerated femoral hernia is treated nonoperatively, and time is wasted with fruitless diagnostic procedures, perforation and peritonitis will result.
5. **C** Indirect inguinal hernia is most common in both males and females, although femoral is relatively more frequent in females.
6. **C** Aberrant obturator artery arising from external instead of internal iliac artery may be lacerated.
7. **A** Hence, *routine* barium enema is not recommended.
8. **D** The inguinal ligament forms the inferior border of Hesselbach's triangle and the superior border of the femoral triangle.
9. **E** The external ring is irrelevant in inguinal hernia repair.
10. **B**
11. **E**
12. **C**
13. **A**
14. **D**

16. Small Intestine

ANATOMY

Vascular Supply
1. Arterial from superior mesenteric artery—best supply to mesenteric border—hence, ischemia affects antimesenteric side first
2. Venous to superior mesenteric vein → portal vein
3. Lymph to mesenteric lymphatics (some from Peyer's patches in submucosa) → regional lymph nodes → cisterna chyli

Histology
1. Mucosa—convoluted to increase surface area by:
   a. Plicae circulares—visible to naked eye
   b. Villi—seen on microscopic examination
   c. Microvilli—seen by electron microscopy; these form the brush border of the columnar cells and are responsible for absorption
      i. The Crypts of Lieberkühn = proliferating, undifferentiated cells, phagocytes
2. Submucosa
   a. *The strongest layer → must be included in intestinal sutures*
   b. Contains nerve edings:
      i. Parasympathetic—from right vagus
      ii. Splanchnic sympathetics—sensitive to distention
3. Muscularis
   a. Inner circular
   b. Outer longitudinal
4. Serosa—outermost layer

INTESTINAL OBSTRUCTION

CLASSIFICATION

1. Simple obstruction: no vascular compromise
2. Strangulating obstruction: associated vascular obstruction, necrosis occurs in three to four hours, especially in pure venous obstruction; difficult to diagnose preoperatively
3. Paralytic (adynamic) ileus: impairment of muscle function

4. Closed-loop obstruction: blockage at two points; vomiting will not help to decrease building pressure in that segment

ETIOLOGY

Small Bowel
1. Adhesions—71 percent
   a. Secondary to previous operation (usually pelvic)
   b. Secondary to inflammatory process
   c. Pathogenesis
      i. Trauma to peritoneal surfaces
      ii. Foreign material (glove powder)
      iii. Devascularization
      iv. Eosinophil deficiency(?)
2. Hernia
   a. Internal—2.5 percent
   b. External—6 percent
3. Tumors—9 percent
   a. Primary
   b. Seeding of metastases in peritoneum
4. Inflammatory disease (Crohn's)—3.7 percent
5. Midgut volvulus (usually neonatal)
6. Intussusception
   a. Usually under age two
   b. If older, look for polyp at apex of intussusception
7. Obturator obstruction
   a. Gallstone ileus
   b. Bezoar
   c. Foreign body
8. Vascular obstruction (mesenteric thrombosis)

Large Bowel
1. Carcinoma (two-thirds visible by sigmoidoscope)
2. Diverticulitis
3. Volvulus
   a. Sigmoid
   b. Cecum
4. Left inguinal hernia with sigmoid incarceration
5. Metastatic carcinoma
6. Congenital bands
7. Inferior mesenteric artery occlusion
8. Segmental vasculitis

CLINICAL MANIFESTATIONS

Small Bowel
1. High-pitched bowel sounds
2. Vomiting—earlier with higher obstruction

3. Fecal vomiting—after three days of obstruction of ileum
4. Distention—more with lower obstruction
5. Obstipation
6. Loss of electrolytes
7. Stepladder pattern of differential air/fluid levels on x-ray with no colonic gas

Large Bowel
1. Little vomiting (less with competent ileocecal valve, *rarely* fecal)
2. Little loss of electrolytes
3. Distention (severe)
4. Constipation and obstipation
5. X-ray shows gas-filled colon to point of obstruction
6. Rectal—obstructing lesion palpable in most cases

Paralytic Ileus
1. Silent abdomen
2. X-ray shows gas in colon and small bowel with identical air/fluid levels (See Fig. 16-1)

COMPLICATIONS

Small Bowel
1. Dehydration
2. Uremia
3. Shock
4. Prolonged distention → mucosal ischemia → release of toxins
5. Strangulation → necrosis → perforation → peritonitis

Large Bowel
1. Cecal perforation (closed loop obstruction if competent ileocecal valve)
2. Strangulation → necrosis → perforation → peritonitis

THERAPY

Small bowel
1. Intravenous fluids; monitoring
2. Operation
   a. Indications
      i. Peritoneal signs
      ii. No improvement in 24 hours
      iii. Some advocate immediate operation after hydration
   b. Procedure
      i. Decompress aseptically intraoperatively with Leonard tube (peroral) if very distended
      ii. Lyse all adhesions; resect pathology

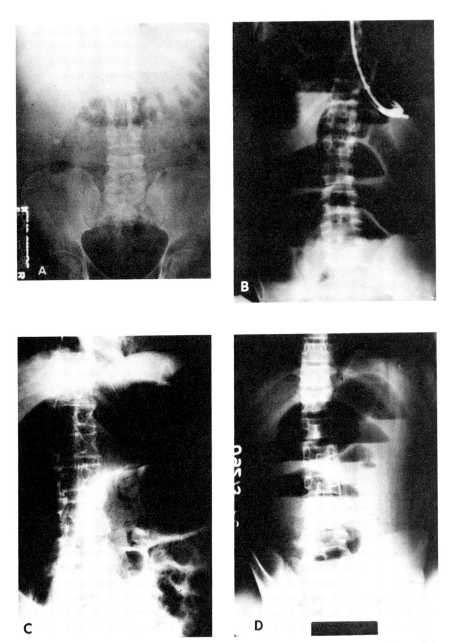

Figure 16-1 Upright film of normal abdomen (A), small bowel obstruction with multiple differential air/fluid levels (B), colonic obstruction due to sigmoid volvulus (C), and postoperative adynamic ileus (D).

   iii. Prevention of recurrent obstruction due to adhesions (debated)
      1) Noble plication (many complications)
      2) Transmesenteric plication (Childs-Phillips). Plicate mesentery to form accordion-like pleats of small bowel and mesentery
      3) Baker tube ("stitchless") plication—use long tube through jejunostomy as a stent for at least 10 days
3. In selected cases of early postoperative or recurrent obstruction, a trial of long tube (Kantor or Miller-Abbott) decompression may be of value

Large Bowel
1. Nasogastric tube
2. Intravenous fluids, antibiotics
3. Barium enema—may reduce intussusception
4. Proctosigmoidoscopy—to reduce sigmoid volvulus
5. Operation; resection with or without preliminary decompressive colostomy or cecostomy (see under specific conditions)

MORTALITY INCREASED BY:

1. Inadequate correction of fluid and electrolyte deficiencies
2. Presence of strangulation obstruction
3. Delays in operative intervention
4. Intraoperative peritoneal soilage
5. Vomiting with aspiration during anesthesia

DETERMINATION OF VIABILITY OF BOWEL

1. Return of normal color
2. Arterial pulsations
3. Peristalsis
4. Thermocouple to determine "reactive hyperemia;" sterile Doppler probe(?)

NEOPLASMS

INCIDENCE

1. 3 percent of all gastrointestinal tumors
2. 1 percent of all malignant tumors
3. Average age 56
4. M > F

CLINICAL FINDINGS (in decreasing order of frequency)

1. Weight loss
2. Abdominal pain
3. Anemia
4. Nausea/vomiting
5. Diarrhea/constipation
6. Bleeding (usually melena)
7. Abdominal mass
8. Obstruction
9. Jaundice

Note: Asymptomatic—6 percent of malignant tumors, 50 percent of benign tumors

DIAGNOSIS

1. Often made only at laparotomy
2. Small bowel series—antegrade or retrograde
3. Endoscopy
4. Selective visceral arteriography—especially for bleeding

PATHOLOGY

Malignant
1. Adenocarcinoma: most common; usually located near ligament of Treitz
2. Malignant carcinoid: usually in ileum
3. Leiomyosarcoma
4. Lymphoma, reticulum cell sarcoma, or Hodgkin's disease
5. Metastatic, especially melanoma

Benign
1. Adenoma
2. Leiomyoma
3. Lipoma
4. Benign carcinoid
5. Hamartoma
6. Villous adenoma (usually in duodenum, premalignant)
7. Vascular tumors (or malformations)
   a. Try to identify bleeding point on angiogram preoperatively
   b. Otherwise, may use methylene blue intraoperatively
   c. Confirm removal by specimen arteriography

Second Primary Tumors
1. About 18 percent of patients with small bowel tumors will be found to have tumors in other organs

TREATMENT

For Cure
1. Wide resection of bowel and mesentery
2. Tumor in duodenum—Whipple procedure
3. Tumor in distal ileum—include right hemicolectomy
4. Postoperative radiotherapy—debated

For Palliation
1. Bypass alone

PROGNOSIS

Five-year Survival Rate
1. Adenocarcinoma 20 percent
2. Lymphoma 40 percent
3. Leiomyosarcoma 50 percent
4. Carcinoid 50 percent

Note: Poor survival statistics relate to lack of clinical suspicion with relatively late diagnosis

PEUTZ-JEGHERS SYNDROME

1. Definition: mucocutaneous pigmentation; hamartomas of small bowel; inherited as autosomal dominant
2. Malignant potential: slight tendency to develop coexistent gastric, small and large bowel malignancies; hamartomas themselves are not premalignant
3. Management:
   a. Differentiate from other forms of gastrointestinal polyposis (familial polyposis and Gardner's syndrome affect mainly colon, are adenomatous and highly premalignant)
   b. Operate only for bleeding or obstruction (intussusception); then excise offending lesions and all lesions over 2 cm; use enterotomy and polypectomy or conservative resection
   c. Pay particular attention to stomach, duodenum, and colon in young patients

RADIATION INJURY

Etiology
1. Progressive obliterative vasculitis
2. Hence, aggravated by hypertension, diabetes, and atherosclerosis
3. Duration from radiation to first operation for injury averages 18 months

Usual Pathology
1. Small bowel—obstruction
2. Colon—bleeding
3. Rectum—obstruction or fistula

Therapy
1. Try *not* to lyse adhesions
2. Resection or bypass with wide margins
   a. Confirm viability by frozen section of margins
   b. Problems with resection include:
      i. Division of mesenteric vessels to already ischemic bowel
      ii. Extensive mobilization may be required
3. Exteriorization, if uncertain about viability

Nonoperative Management
(Try to manage patients with minimal symptoms or with proctitis nonoperatively)
1. Low-residue diet
2. Sedation and antispasmodics
3. Stool softeners
4. Steroid enemas for proctitis
5. Azulfidine (?)
6. Home hyperalimentation for intractable chronic symptoms

Complications of Operative Management
1. Anastomotic leak in about 30 percent
2. Systemic failure
3. Abscesses
4. Wound dehiscence
5. Mortality about 35 percent

DIVERTICULAR DISEASE OF JEJUNUM

Location
1. Usually proximal
2. Mesenteric border between leaves of mesentery
3. Most are multiple, false diverticuli

Associated Factors
1. Advanced age
2. Diverticulosis elsewhere
3. Jejunal dyskinesia = intestinal hypermotility and muscular hypertrophy

Clinical Findings
1. Postprandial bloating
2. Cramping pain
3. Weight loss, marked
4. Rare complications include
   a. Obstruction
   b. Bleeding
   c. Perforation
   d. Chronic pneumoperitoneum
   e. Blind-loop syndrome with malabsorption

Diagnosis
1. Usually—incidentally, at laparotomy for something else
2. Occasionally—by barium studies

Therapy
1. Incidentally found diverticuli—no therapy unless bowel is dilated and hypertrophied
2. Otherwise, resection of hypertrophied bowel containing the diverticuli, which may be identified by insufflation of 50-100 cc air into upper small bowel
3. If operation contraindicated for medical reasons,
   a. Low-residue diet
   b. Frequent small meals
   c. Antispasmodics
   d. Rest supine for 1 hour after eating
   e. Intermittent courses of oral antibiotics for blind-loop syndrome

---

MECKEL'S DIVERTICULUM

▶ **Description ("Rule of Twos"): remnant of omphalomesenteric duct—a true diverticulum found on antimesenteric border of ileum**
1. Usually *two* feet from ileocecal valve
2. Usually about *two* inches long
3. Occurs in *two* percent of population
4. *Two* types of heterotropic mucosa:
   a. Gastric—may cause ulceration in adjacent ileum or within diverticulum—massive bleeding, especially in children
   b. Pancreatic
   c. Rarely, other types of heterotopic mucosa

Pathology
1. Diverticulitis—usually misdiagnosed as appendicitis
2. Bleeding—diagnose by 99m Technetium scan—taken up by parietal cells in heterotopic gastric mucosa, if present

3. Intestinal obstruction—by entrapment, volvulus or intussusception
4. Neoplasms—rare

Therapy
1. Excision
2. If found incidentally at laparotomy for another reason, excision debated

ACUTE MESENTERIC ISCHEMIA

Clinical Findings
1. Early lack of objective findings
2. Severe generalized abdominal pain—out of proportion to signs
3. Nausea, vomiting, diarrhea, constipation—variable
4. Later: tenderness, distention, peritonitis, shock

Diagnosis
1. Laboratory findings include
   a. Heme-positive stool
   b. Severe leukocytosis
   c. Increased serum amylase
   d. Base deficits
2. Plain x-ray
   a. Air/fluid levels in dilated bowel
   b. Blunt plicae
   c. Thickened, edematous bowel wall
   d. Intramural and portal gas—late finding
3. Barium studies—"thumbprinting," disordered motility
4. Mesenteric angiography—for evaluation of larger vessels only

Therapy

Most Important is Early Operation—Even Without Confirmatory Studies
1. Massive volume replacement, antibiotics, anticoagulants, bicarbonate
2. *For venous infarction,* resect involved bowel and treat underlying process:
   a. Hypercoagulability
   b. Portal hypertension
   c. Sepsis
3. *For arterial infarction,*
   a. Open occluded vessel—bypass or endarterectomy better than thrombectomy alone
   b. Then resect nonviable bowel, but do *not* anastomose
   c. Second-look laparotomy at 6 to 12 hours, at which time anastomosis may be performed if bowel is viable

Prognosis
1. Only 30 percent survival

MORBID OBESITY

COMPLICATIONS

1. Hypertension
2. Diabetes mellitus
3. Hyperlipidemia
4. Pickwickian syndrome
5. Cardiac disease, etc.

INDICATIONS FOR SURGERY

1. Failure of medical and psychiatric therapy, *and*
2. At least twice ideal weight (or over 100 pounds above ideal weight), *and*
3. Emotionally stable and well-informed patient
4. Presence of complications of obesity

TECHNIQUES

Gastric Bypass or Gastric Staple Plication
1. Technique: leave 10 percent gastric remnant
2. Mechanism of weight loss: eats less
3. Complications: many fewer than intestinal bypass; but technically more difficult procedure

Jejunoileal Bypass
1. "14-to-4"
   a. Jejunum 14 inches (35 cm) from ligament of Treitz anastomosed *end-to-side* to ileum 4 inches (10 cm) from ileocecal valve
   b. Reflux into bypassed segment may allow absorption and cause failure of operation
   c. *End-to-end* anastomosis prevents reflux. In this operation, distal end is anastomosed to the colon
2. Weight loss
   a. 10 pounds per month for first six months
   b. This is due to
      i. Malabsorption
      ii. Eating less because of diarrhea
3. Complications
   a. Operative mortality 2 to 6 percent

b. Diarrhea, steatorrhea, flatulence
c. Crampy pain
d. Electrolyte imbalance: hypokalemia or hypocalcemia
e. Impaired absorption of: fat, cholesterol, and vitamins A, D, K
f. Loss of body cell mass in addition to fat
g. Oxalate urinary tract calculi
h. Polyarthritis, gout
i. Colonic dilatation
j. Hepatic steatosis (in most patients at first)
k. Cirrhosis, liver failure
   i. Etiology
     1) Protein malnutrition
     2) Endotoxins from bacterial overgrowth in bypassed segment
     3) Psychogenic vomiting (?)
     4) Lithocholic acid (breakdown product of unabsorbed bile acids in colon) is hepatotoxic
   ii. Diagnosis
     1) Needle liver biopsy
     2) R/O common duct stones
   iii. Prevention: patients must not use alcohol
   iv. Treatment: take down bypass
l. Bypass enteropathy
   i. Etiology: bacterial proliferation
   ii. Clinical findings: diarrhea, distention, fever, pain
   iii. Treatment
     1) Antibiotics (Vibramycin for Bacteroides)
     2) Jejunostomy with proximal end of bypassed segment for feeding if necessary
m. Complications requiring take down of bypass occur in 10 to 20 percent of patients

BYPASS FOR HYPERLIPIDEMIA

1. Indications: still experimental
2. Technique: bypass distal one-third (200 cm) of distal ileum
3. Result
   a. Serum cholesterol decreases by 50 percent
   b. Total body cholesterol decreases by 33 percent
   c. Plasma triglycerides decrease by 50 percent in primary hypertriglyceridemia
4. Mechanism
   a. Reduced absorption
   b. Increased hepatic synthesis of bile salts from cholesterol to compensate for fecal losses
5. Result: remission or improvement in angina pectoris in 67 percent

SELECTED BIBLIOGRAPHY

Buchwald H: Morbid obesity. Surg Clin North Am 59(6): December 1979

Herbsman H, Wetstein L, Rosen Y, et al.: Tumors of the small intestine. Curr Probl Surg 17(3): March 1980

Nadrowski LF: Pathophysiology and current treatment of intestinal obstruction. Rev Surg 31:381, 1974

Rosato EF: Intestinal obstruction. In Brooks FP (ed): Gastrointestinal Pathophysiology. London, Oxford Univ Press, 1974

QUESTIONS

A 40-year-old female complains of nausea, vomiting, and obstipation of 48 hours duration. She is noted to be moderately distended and to have high-pitched bowel sounds. Abdominal upright film shows a stepladder small bowel pattern of differential air/fluid levels.

1. If she has had previous surgery, it was most likely:
   A. Cholecystectomy
   B. Gastric
   C. Pelvic
   D. Small bowel resection
   E. Hernia repair
2. Reliable indications ruling out strangulated small bowel obstruction include:
   A. Absence of fever and leukocytosis
   B. Normal plain film of the abdomen
   C. Lack of peritoneal signs
   D. All of these
   E. None of these
3. Most reliable in determining bowel viability during laparotomy is return of:
   A. Normal color
   B. Peristalsis
   C. Mesenteric arterial pulsations
   D. Normal temperature
   E. Mesenteric venous flow
4. The use of antihistamines in prevention of postoperative adhesions is based on the observation that areas of adhesion formation appear to *lack:*
   A. Fibroblastic proliferation
   B. Mast cells
   C. Lymphocytes
   D. Eosinophils
   E. Capillary dilatation
5. Currently, prevention of postoperative adhesions is best accomplished in practice by:
   A. Transmesenteric plication
   B. Stitchless plication
   C. Careful closure of all serosal surfaces
   D. Careful closure of the parietal peritoneum
   E. None of these

6. A 70-year-old female with generalized atherosclerosis complains of severe diffuse abdominal pain for the past two hours. Her stool is Hematest-positive and blood gases are pH-7.23, pO_2=68, pCO_2=19. Physical examination reveals no peritoneal signs and the abdominal flat plate is within normal limits. Appropriate therapy after correction of the acid-based abnormality is:
   A. Gastroscopy
   B. Upper GI series
   C. Barium enema
   D. Laparotomy
   E. Angiography

7. Concerning the small intestine, which of the following is most likely to cause pain?
   A. Direct application of cautery
   B. Cutting with a scalpel
   C. Crushing with a clamp
   D. Distention
   E. Application of a chemical irritant to the serosa

8. The *least* common site of gastrointestinal cancer is the:
   A. Oral cavity
   B. Esophagus
   C. Stomach
   D. Small bowel
   E. Rectum

9. The operative procedure of choice for resectable periampullary cancer involves removing a portion of each of the following structures *except:*
   A. Stomach
   B. Duodenum
   C. Common bile duct
   D. Portal vein
   E. Pancreas

10. Which of the following conditions involving the small intestine is most likely to be associated with malignancy?
   A. Peutz-Jeghers syndrome
   B. Gardner's syndrome
   C. Juvenile (retention) polyps
   D. Hereditory hemorrhagic telangiectasia (Osler-Weber-Rendu syndrome)
   E. Crohn's disease

11. An 80-year-old female complains of intermittent postprandial epigastric pain and constipation alternating with flatulence. She has lost 30 pounds over the past four months. On physical examination there is an abdominal bruit and heme-positive stool. Upper gastrointestinal series, barium enema, gastroscopy, proctoscopy, and colonoscopy are within normal limits. Of the following, the laboratory study most likely to be diagnostic is:
   A. Endoscopic retrograde cholangiopancreatography
   B. Arteriography
   C. Venography
   D. Sonography
   E. Intravenous pyelography

12. A 70-year-old male who has had intermittent episodes of midabdominal
    pain, especially after eating, comes to your office complaining that the pain
    has become more constant over the last two hours. On examination, you
    find him to have a mildly distended abdomen with mild tenderness
    throughout, but no peritoneal signs. On rectal examination, Hematest-
    positive stool is found. His white cell count is 29,000 and he appears
    diaphoretic. Appropriate management at this point would be:
    A. Intravenous hydration, exploratory laparotomy
    B. Proctoscopy and barium enema
    C. Upper gastrointestinal series
    D. Nonoperative management for acute pancreatitis
    E. Endoscopic retrograde cholangiopancreatography
13. Complications of jejunoileal bypass for morbid obesity do *not* include:
    A. Steatorrhea
    B. Oxalate urinary tract calculi
    C. Scurvy
    D. Hypocalcemia
    E. Gout
14. Jejunoileal bypass for hyperlipidemia differs from that for morbid obesity in:
    A. Frequency of steatorrhea postoperatively
    B. Amount of postoperative weight loss
    C. Incidence of nephrolithiasis
    D. Operative procedure
    E. All of these

ANSWERS

1. **C**
2. **E** Less than one of three are diagnosed correctly preoperatively—there are
        no *reliable* signs *ruling out* strangulation obstruction before exploration.
3. **B** However, newer tests such as 99m Technetium-tagged albumin
        microspheres, EMG, and thermocouples are promising advances in
        determining bowel viability intraoperatively.
4. **D** The theory is that antihistamine activity of eosinophils decreases the role
        of mast-cell-induced inflammation.
5. **E** Intestinal plication prevents recurrent intestinal obstruction due to
        adhesions—not adhesions themselves. Closure of serosal and parietal
        surfaces, contrary to previous thought, do not appear to diminish
        adhesions. In all, only elimination of talc from gloves has led to
        significant diminution of postoperative adhesions.
6. **D** A pattern of abdominal pain with minimal abdominal findings and
        metabolic acidosis in an elderly patient with atherosclerosis should raise
        a high suspicion of occlusion of the superior mesenteric artery leading to
        infarction of the small bowel. No time should be wasted in bringing
        these patients to the operating room, because their only hope for
        survival is early exploration and removal of the thrombus before

gangrene of the whole small bowel occurs. The superior mesenteric artery provides blood supply from the ligament of Treitz to the mid-transverse colon, and so complete infarction of this segment of bowel is incompatible with life. Anticoagulation should be initiated on suspicion of this condition.

7. **D** Visceral pain is due to distention. It is perfectly possible to perform minor operations on the bowel (such as jejunostomy) if local anesthesia is applied as the parietal peritoneum is entered, without any anesthesia of the visceral peritoneum. On the other hand, the *parietal* peritoneum is sensitive to cutting, crushing, heat, or chemical irritation.

8. **D** The small intestine is a very uncommon site of malignancy. Late diagnosis makes it a very lethal lesion.

9. **D** The procedure of choice for periampullary cancer is pancreatico-duodenectomy (Whipple procedure). This entails removing the distal stomach, common bile duct, gallbladder, duodenum, and the pancreas to midbody. Truncal vagotomy is also performed to alleviate peptic ulceration. The portal vein is dissected free of the pancreas and preserved.

10. **B** Gardner's syndrome is an autosomal dominant heridatary condition characterized by multiple adenomatous polyps of the colon and sometimes small bowel. In addition, these patients have osteomas and sebaceous cysts of the skin and subcutaneous tissue. The polyps of Gardner's syndrome commonly become adenocarcinomas. Peutz-Jeghers syndrome includes hamartomas of the small bowel that are not premalignant, and operation is indicated only for symptoms. Juvenile (retention) polyps are more common in the colon but do occur in the small bowel. They autoamputate before puberty and operation is indicated only for bleeding or obstruction. Osler-Weber-Rendu syndrome is an inborn progressive tendency toward formation of dilated endothelial spaces in the small bowel and other sites, causing vascular malformations and hemangiomas that may bleed or cause intussusception. Crohn's disease, which usually involves the terminal ileum, virtually never gives rise to malignancy, and operation is indicated only for complications or intractability.

11. **B** This is a typical case of abdominal angina due to stenosis of a mesenteric artery (usually superior, sometimes celiac). Diagnosis is made by arteriography, and vascular reconstruction may be possible.

12. **A** This is another patient who probably has a mesenteric infarction. The key is previous episodes of midabdominal pain after eating (chronic mesenteric insufficiency) and then a distended abdomen, heme-positive stool, and high white count. Pancreatitis may be a possibility; however, an amalyse of only 450 and blood in his stool make this much less likely.

13. **C** Jejunoileal bypass for morbid obesity leads to malabsorption of fat, cholesterol, vitamins A, D, and K. Vitamin C absorption is normal.

14. **E** For hyperlipidemia, only the distal one third of the small intestine is bypassed. Weight loss may not occur. Other complications are also lessened.

17. Appendix

ANATOMY

1. Base—posteromedial aspect of cecum below ileocecal valve
2. Free end—may be in numerous locations: pelvic, retrocecal, retroileal, LLQ, RLQ, paracolic (See Fig. 17-1)
3. Teniae of colon—converge at base of appendix

PHYSIOLOGY

1. Lymphoid organ (tonsils, Peyer's patches, appendix are all immunologic analogues of the avian bursa of Fabricius—responsible for immunoglobulin production)

ETIOLOGY OF APPENDICITIS

Closed loop obstruction of lumen (by fecalith, lymphoid hypertrophy, barium inspissation, seeds, worms)
↓ Mucous secretion into lumen
Distention (*vague midabdominal pain*—visceral pain)
↓
Peristalsis (*crampy pain*)
↓
Multiplication of bacteria (toxins cause *fever, tachycardia, and leukocytosis*)
↓
Distention exceeds venous pressure
↓ *Nausea and vomiting*
Vascular congestion
↓
Serosal inflammation (*RLQ parietal pain*)
↓
Perforation

INCIDENCE

1. 7 percent lifetime chance of developing appendicitis

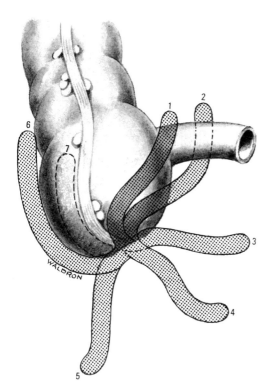

Figure 17-1 Variations in the location of the appendix: preileal (1), postileal (2), promontoric (3), pelvic (4), subcecal (5), paracolic (6), retrocecal (7). *(From Maingot R (ed):* Abdominal Operations, *6th Edt. Appleton-Century-Crofts, 1974, 1352, with permission.)*

CLINICAL FINDINGS

1. Pain
2. Anorexia (almost always)
3. Vomiting (75 percent)
4. Obstipation
5. Diarrhea (especially retrocecal)
6. Tenderness (McBurney's point, or on rectal if retrocecal)
7. Cutaneous hyperesthesia
8. Guarding, rebound

Confirmatory Signs
1. Rovsing's sign—RLQ pain on palpation of LLQ
2. Psoas sign—stretch of psoas muscle elicits pain
3. Obturator sign—stretch of obturator internus

LABORATORY FINDINGS

1. White cell count 10,000 to 18,000 (10 percent have normal WBC)
2. Urinalysis—no bacteria, occasional hematuria, especially with retrocecal appendix

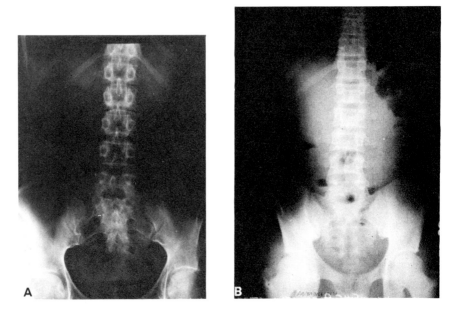

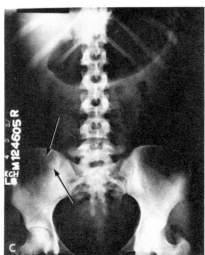

Figure 17-2 Abdominal flat plates. Normal (A), air/fluid levels in right lower quadrant due to appendicitis, (B), and fecaliths in inflamed appendix (C).

X-RAY FINDINGS (See Fig. 17-2)

1. Fecalith (diagnostic if present)
2. Air/fluid levels in RLQ
3. Altered right psoas shadow

DIFFERENTIAL DIAGNOSIS

1. Acute mesenteric lymphadenitis
2. No organic pathology
3. Acute pelvic inflammatory disease
4. Twisted ovarian cyst
5. Ruptured Graffian follicle
6. Acute gastroenteritis
7. Meckel's diverticulitis
8. Urinary tract infection
9. Intussusception
10. Regional enteritis
11. Primary peritonitis
12. Henoch-Schonlein purpura
13. Endometriosis
14. Ruptured ectopic pregnancy
15. Torsion testis
16. Acute epididymitis
17. Others

THERAPY

1. Appendectomy: incision may be McBurney (oblique muscle splitting) or transverse (for cosmetic reasons). Drain if localized abscess and use delayed skin closure
2. Expectant therapy (Ochsner): if abscess diagnosed preoperatively, may treat with NG suction and antibiotics, then elective appendectomy. This is controversial

COMPLICATIONS

1. Perforation (usually not within 12 hours of onset of symptoms)
2. Peritonitis
3. Abscess
4. Pyelphlebitis
   a. Suppurative thrombophlebitis of the portal system
   b. Shaking chills, fever, jaundice
   c. Air may be seen within portal system
   d. Rare, but grave, complication

PROGNOSIS

Mortality
1. Unruptured 0.1 percent
2. Ruptured 3 percent

Aim in Improvement of Mortality
1. High index of suspicion → 15 to 20 percent negative laparotomy rate acceptable

TUMORS OF APPENDIX

Incidence
1. 1.4 percent of appendectomies

Types
1. Carcinoid
   a. Usually benign
   b. 3 percent metastasize to nodes
   c. Carcinoid syndrome rare—due to hepatic metastases
   d. Usually simple appendectomy is sufficient therapy for small carcinoid
2. Adenocarcinoma
   a. Requires right hemicolectomy
   b. 10 percent have widespread metastases when discovered
3. Mucocele
   a. Usually benign
   b. However, rupture may result in pseudomyxoma peritonei

SELECTED BIBLIOGRAPHY

Fee HJ, et al.: Radiologic diagnosis of appendicitis. Arch Surg 112:742, 1977
Lewis FR, et al.: Appendicitis: A critical review of diagnosis and treatment in 1000 cases. Arch Surg 110:677, 1975

QUESTIONS

A 22-year-old male with a temperature of 102°F and right lower quadrant tenderness is explored through a McBurney incision and found to have acute appendicitis with perforation at the base. It is thought that removal of the appendix will leave a large defect in the inflamed cecal wall.
1. The procedure of choice is:
   A. Appendectomy and closure of the defect with heavy silk sutures tied tightly
   B. Appendectomy and closure of the defect with an omental patch
   C. Cecectomy
   D. Right hemicolectomy
   E. Appendectomy and tube cecostomy
2. Six days postoperatively, the patient develops severe, shaking chills with fever, cyanosis, profuse sweating, and appears jaundiced. The most likely diagnosis is:
   A. Gram-negative septicemia
   B. Serum hepatitis

    C. Ascending cholangitis
    D. Pyelonephritis
    E. Pyelphlebitis

3. The most valid reason for *not* performing an incidental appendectomy during cholecystectomy is:
    A. Difficult exposure of the cecum
    B. Probability of fecal fistula
    C. Resultant predisposition to colon cancer
    D. Resultant immunologic defect
    E. Prolonged anesthesia time

4. Exploration through a McBurney incision reveals a normal appendix. Appendectomy alone is the procedure of choice in the event of the discovery of each of the following conditions *except:*
    A. Right salpingitis
    B. Mesenteric adenitis
    C. Regional enteritis involving the cecum
    D. Retrocecal appendix
    E. No intraabdominal pathology

5. Pathological report of an incidental appendectomy specimen reveals a small carcinoid tumor of the tip of the appendix without involvement of mesentery. Appropriate therapy should include:
    A. Cecectomy
    B. Right hemicolectomy
    C. Reexploration with mesenteric node biopsy
    D. Chemotherapy
    E. No further therapy

6. The most frequent site of carcinoid tumor is the:
    A. Jejunum
    B. Liver
    C. Ileum
    D. Appendix
    E. Colon

7. The least likely finding in acute retrocecal appendicitis is:
    A. Normal white cell count
    B. Lack of point tenderness at McBurney's point
    C. Bacteriuria
    D. Hematuria
    E. Diarrhea

8. Least likely etiologic agent in acute appendicitis:
    A. High-fiber diet
    B. Fecalith
    C. Barium inspissation
    D. Lymphoid hypertrophy
    E. Foreign body in appendix

9. An 18-year-old female on exploration for suspected acute appendicitis is found to have a mildly inflamed right fallopian tube and a normal appendix. The appropriate operative procedure would be:
    A. Appendectomy and right salpingectomy

   B. Right salpingectomy
   C. Bilateral salpingectomy
   D. Appendectomy
   E. Close without removing any organ

ANSWERS

1. **E** Cecostomy may be performed if a large cecal defect remains after appendectomy. Attempts to close such defects may result in unwanted fecal fistula or abscess.

2. **E** Other findings in pyelphlebitis include tender liver, cutaneous petechiae. The prognosis is grave.

3. **A** Although there is still debate, it appears that earlier studies linking appendectomy to future colonic carcinoma were incorrect. Incidental appendectomy is debated, but certainly indicated when appendicoliths are noted. It should not be attempted if exposure is difficult.

4. **C** If Crohn's disease is found to involve the base of the appendix, appendectomy may result in fistula and should, therefore, not be performed. In the other cases listed, appendectomy alone is the procedure of choice.

5. **E** Carcinoid tumors of the appendix usually require no more than simple appendectomy. Exceptions are lesions over 2 cm in diameter, lesions with nodal involvement, or serosal spread.

6. **D** The most common site of carcinoid tumors is the appendix. Hepatic metastases may lead to the carcinoid syndrome. One of 500 appendectomies will reveal carcinoid tumor.

7. **D** Bacteriuria should lead one to suspect urinary tract infection. Hematuria occurs occasionally in appendicitis, especially retrocecal. Ten percent of patients with appendicitis will have a normal white cell count. Diarrhea will sometimes occur in appendicitis, especially retrocecal. Retrocecal appendicitis often requires careful rectal examination to detect tenderness, which may be lacking at McBurney's point.

8. **A** Low-fiber diets may be responsible for a variety of conditions in Western countries. These include hemorrhoids, anal fissures, diverticulitis, and appendicitis.

9. **D** Appendectomy alone is the appropriate treatment when mild salpingitis is found. Antibiotic therapy should then be instituted.

18. Colon, Rectum, and Anus

CANCER

INCIDENCE

1. Second only to skin
2. Synchronous—5 percent
3. Metachronous—2.5 percent
4. Adenocarcinoma—95 percent

ETIOLOGY

1. Genetic predisposition (2 to 3 times)
2. Immunologic deficiency
3. Chronic ulcerative colitis (or granulomatous colitis ?)
4. Low-fiber diet (→ higher concentration of carcinogens in fecal mass)
5. Bacterial dehydrogenation of bile salts (?)

SPREAD

1. Direct extension—encircles bowel and spreads to adjacent organs
2. Hematogenous: Portal vein → liver. Lumbar and vertebral veins → lungs
3. Regional lymph nodes—most common (50 percent of specimens)
4. Gravitational seeding—rectovesical or rectouterine pouches (Blumer's shelf), 3 percent to ovary
5. Perineural
6. Intraluminal (responsible for "anastomotic recurrence")

CLINICAL FINDINGS

1. Doubling time is 620 days—hence, may grow silently for years
2. Clinical findings vary with exact location
   a. Right colon—lesions fungate to large size before diagnosed by
      i. Iron deficiency anemia
      ii. Gross blood in stool

      iii. Vague abdominal pain
      iv. Palpable mass
   b. Left colon—semisolid feces, hence
      i. Alternating constipation and increased frequency of defecation
      ii. Partial obstruction
      iii. Stool streaked with blood or mucus
   c. Rectum
      i. Blood-streaked stool
      ii. Tenesmus
      iii. Feeling of incomplete defecation
   d. In general
      i. Hepatomegaly due to metastases
      ii. Portal obstruction
      iii. Groin or supraclavicular lymphadenopathy
      iv. Weight loss, cachexia
      v. Obstruction, perforation, hemorrhage

DIAGNOSIS

1. Two-thirds within reach of sigmoidoscope
2. One-third within reach of finger
3. Barium enema: perform even if rectal lesion palpated, to rule out synchronous lesion. Shows "apple core" defect, loss of mucosal pattern, inflexible bowel wall
4. Colonoscopy: if barium enema negative, but suspicion high
5. CEA (Carcinoembryonic antigen): glycoprotein in fetal tissues also found in gastrointestinal tumors. Current application is in screening for and confirming recurrent tumor.
6. IVP: to rule out ureteral obstruction in patients to have colon resection

Note: Barium never given orally if left colon tumor since it may precipitate obstruction

THERAPY

1. Wide excision with regional lymph drainage, even if metastases have occurred, for prevention of obstruction or hemorrhage
2. "No-touch" technique
   a. Tie blood vessels
   b. Tie bowel proximal and distal to lesion
   c. Then mobilize and resect bowel
3. For rectal lesions
   a. Miles procedure (abdominoperineal resection)—lesions < 7 cm from anus
      i. Permanent (end) colostomy
      ii. Complications (35 percent) include: ureteral injury, bladder dysfunction, bladder injury

b. Anterior resection—lesions from > 15 cm from anus
   i. Must resect distal margin or 5 cm normal bowel and 10 cm of proximal normal bowel
   ii. Anastomosis below peritoneal reflection
c. If low anterior resection difficult but tumor too high to require abdominoperineal resection (i.e., 7–15 cm) anastomosis may be done:
   i. With anorectal stump everted to facilitate low anastomosis (pull-through procedure), or
   ii. Using end-to-end anastomoring (EEA) stapler
   iii. Problem—sphincter function may not be satisfactory postop
d. Fulguration
   i. Aggressive electrocautery
   ii. Only for lesions below pelvic reflection
   iii. Problem—nodes are not removed
   iv. Application—poor risk patients
e. Radiation therapy—for poor risk patients; or adjuvant
f. Chemotherapy—mainly 5-fluorouracil
4. Treatment of complications
a. Obstruction—alternatives are
   i. Primary resection and anastomosis (usually for right colon)
   ii. Decompression by colostomy or cecostomy, then later resection (usually for left colon)
b. Perforation
   i. Usually Hartmann procedure (resection, proximal colostomy, distal end closed)
   ii. Resection, colostomy, and mucous fistula
   iii. In any case, local drainage and antibiotics
c. Extension—resect other organs en bloc

Dukes classification

Class	Definition	5-year survival rate
A	Bowel wall involvement only	95%
B	Through bowel wall	65%
C	Lymph nodes positive	30%
D	Metastases or unresectable lesion	5%

POLYPS

CLINICAL FINDINGS

1. Rectal bleeding
2. Hypokalemia and mucus in stool (especially villous adenoma)
3. Prolapse through anus

4. Tenesmus, constipation, increased frequency, peristaltic cramps, intussusception (large lesions)

DIAGNOSIS

1. Barium enema—round filling defect with smooth edges
2. Colonoscopy or sigmoidoscopy

TREATMENT

1. Excision via endoscope if small or pedunculated
2. Laparotomy—if endoscopic removal unsuccessful, if large (> 1.5 cm) lesion, or many small lesions
3. If polyp found to contain malignancy, colon resection advisable if:
   a. Invasion through muscularis mucosae into stroma
   b. Lymphatics in head of polyp contain tumor
   c. Tumor near resection margin

PATHOLOGY

1. Adenomatous polyp 60 percent
2. Villous adenoma 10 percent
3. Mixed polyp 15 percent
4. Cancer in adenoma 6 percent
5. Others 9 percent

SYNDROMES ASSOCIATED WITH COLONIC POLYPS

1. Familial polyposis
   a. Autosomal dominant
   b. Adenomatous polyps
   c. Malignancy in *all* patients by age 40
   d. Therapy
      i. Total colectomy and ileorectal anastomosis
      ii. Close follow-up of rectum
2. Gardner's syndrome
   a. Same as above + desmoid tumors, osteomas of skull or mandible, and sebaceous cysts
3. Juvenile polyps
   a. Found in children
   b. Usually autoamputate at puberty
   c. No malignant potential
   d. Familial incidence

  e. Operate only for bleeding or intussusception
4. Peutz-Jeghers syndrome
  a. Autosomal dominant
  b. Polyps of stomach, small bowel, and colon
  c. Melanin spots of skin and mucous membranes
  d. Pathology: hamartomas
  e. No malignant potential
  f. Operate only for complications
5. Pseudopolyposis
  a. Found in ulcerative colitis

DIVERTICULAR DISEASE OF THE COLON

ANATOMY

1. False diverticula = herniations of mucosa and submucosa through circular
   muscle (See Fig. 18-1)

ETIOLOGY

1. Low fiber diet → inappropriate segmentation of circular muscle → segmental
   intraluminal hypertension → pulsion diverticulae with hypertrophy of
   muscles

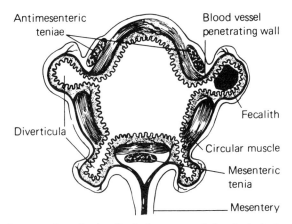

Figure 18-1   Cross section of colon illustrating areas of diverticulosis through defects in circular muscle layer. *(From Dunphy JE and Lay LW (eds):* Current Surgical Diagnosis and Treatment, *3rd Edt. Lange, 1977, p 635, with permission.)*

2. These occur especially where vessels enter colon laterally
3. Morphine causes increased intraluminal pressure
4. Tension = pressure × radius (pressure highest where radius least, e.g., sigmoid)

CLINICAL FINDINGS

1. Asymptomatic (one-fourth to one-half of patients)
2. Hemorrhage
   a. Not associated with diverticulitis
   b. Often profuse, unlike that due to carcinoma
3. Obstruction of neck of "tic" by fecal plug → infection → longitudinal spread → intraluminal fistula (seen on barium enema) → edema obstructing other "tics" → diverticulitis
▶4. "Left-sided appendicitis" (same symptoms as appendicitis, but in LLQ)

DIAGNOSIS

1. Proctoscopy: in diverticulitis, immobility of bowel may prevent insertion greater than 15 cm
2. Barium enema (see Fig. 18-2)
   a. Long segment with gradual transition to normal bowel
   b. Spastic bowel
   c. Picket fence (saw tooth) contour may be early stage of diverticulosis
   d. May find coexistent carcinoma

COMPLICATIONS

1. Obstruction
2. Perforation
3. Fistula to bladder (pneumaturia or fecaluria), uterus, vagina, ileum, or ureter
4. Hemorrhage

MEDICAL THERAPY

1. High-fiber diet (increased radius → decreased pressure)
2. Antispasmodics (such as Probanthine or Bentyl)
3. Bulk laxatives

SURGICAL THERAPY

Indications
1. Severe progressive inflammatory disease
2. Failure of medical management

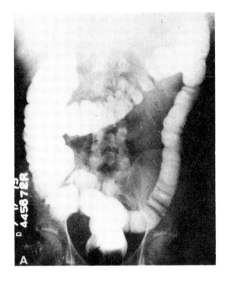
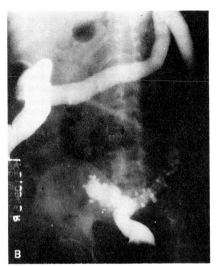
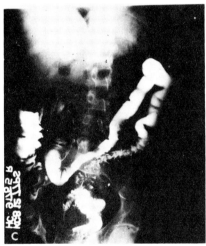

Figure 18-2 Normal barium enema (A), diverticulosis (B) and diverticulitis (C).

3. Stricture (to rule out malignancy)
4. General peritonitis
5. Uncontrollable or recurrent hemorrhage
6. Fistula or perforation

Procedure
1. Hemorrhage (usually ascending colon)
   a. Resect involved segment, or
   b. Total colectomy with ileoproctostomy, or
   c. Resection based on intraoperative colonoscopy or based on arteriographic localization, or

    d. Often nonoperative therapy is sufficient (see below)
2. Peritonitis
    a. Drainage and antibiotics, or
    b. If fecal leak
       i. Diverting colostomy, or
      ii. Exteriorization, or
     iiii. Hartmann procedure
3. Obstruction or fistula
    a. Completely diverting colostomy, then
    b. Resection at a second stage, then
    c. Close colostomy
    d. In some cases (a) and (b) may be performed concurrently, especially if carcinoma suspected
4. Colomyotomy
    a. Split circular muscle of colon through taenia
    b. Results in decreased intraluminal pressure
    c. Indications—uncertain at this time

RADIOLOGIC THERAPY

1. Arteriography
    a. To locate bleeder
    b. With vasopressin (ADH) infusion is 92 percent successful in at least temporarily stopping hemorrhage
2. Barium enema
    a. Effective in tamponading bleeder
    b. Not *prior* to angiogram since barium in colon may interfere

CECAL DIVERTICULA

1. True diverticula (i.e., contain all histologic layers)
2. Rare
3. When inflamed, they mimic appendicitis
4. When asymptomatic, no therapy indicated
5. When inflamed, excise or drain

ULCERATIVE COLITIS

PATHOLOGY

1. Mucosal inflammation
    a. Abscesses in crypts of Liebrkuhn with decreased numbers of Goblet cells
    b. Horizontal spread causing mucosal slough

   c. Intervening normal mucosa → pseudopolyps
   d. Vascular congestion, hemorrhages
2. In advanced cases, full thickness involvement
   a. Colon becomes shortened
   b. Mesentery remains thin (unlike regional enteritis)

INCIDENCE

1. Two peaks: second and sixth decades

PATTERNS OF INVOLVEMENT

1. Rectum alone (ulcerative proctitis)—50 percent
2. Whole colon (pancolitis)—30 percent
3. Backwash ileitis—10 percent of patients with pancolitis

CLINICAL FINDINGS

1. Bloody diarrhea
2. Tenesmus, urgency, incontinence
3. Crampy abdominal pain
4. Fever, weight loss, dehydration

DIAGNOSIS

1. Sigmoidoscopy, colonoscopy: granular, hyperemic, friable mucosa
2. Plain abdominal films: to rule out megacolon
3. Barium enema (See Fig. 18-3)
   a. Findings
      i. Loss of haustral markings
      ii. Pseudopolyposis
      iii. Shortening of colon
      iv. Stricture (watch for malignancy)
   b. Contradictions
      i. Acute disease
      ii. Megacolon

COMPLICATIONS ("*ULCERATIVE COLITIS*")   ◄

Extracolonic
1. Urinary calculi
2. Liver: pericholangitis, cirrhosis, sclerosing cholangitis, carcinoma of the bile
   ducts, fatty infiltration

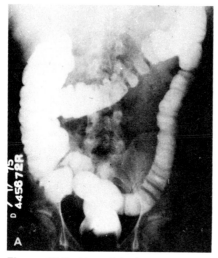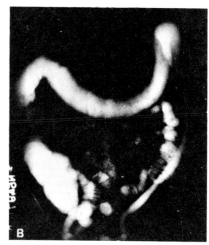

Figure 18-3 Normal barium enema (A) and one showing of colon and loss of haustral markings in ulcerative colitis (B).

3. Cholelithiasis
4. Epithelium: erythema nodosum, erythema multiforme, pyoderma gangrenosum, pustular dermatitis, aphthous stomatitis
5. Retardation of growth and sexual maturation in children
6. Arthralgias, arthritis, ankylosing spondylitis, periarthritis
7. Thrombophlebitis, migratory
8. Iatrogenic: due to steroids, blood transfusions, operations
9. Vitamin deficiencies
10. Eyes: uveitis, chorioretinitis, iridocyclitis

Colonic

1. Cancer
   a. Risk is 3 percent over first 10 years, then 20 percent of population at risk for each subsequent 10 years
   b. Survival rates low due to late detection
   c. Follow with serial rectal biopsy, CEA
   d. Greatest risk of cancer: severe first attack, pancolitis, chronic *continuous* symptoms, early onset
2. Obstruction: unusual
3. Leakage (perforation — 3 percent): most common cause of death
4. Iron deficiency (*hemorrhage*)
5. Toxic megacolon (3 percent)
6. Inanition
7. Stricture, fistulas, perirectal abscesses

MEDICAL THERAPY

1. Bed rest
2. Diet free of milk
3. Correction of anemia and hypokalemia
4. Azulfidine (sulfasalazine) or Gantrisin (sulfisoxazole)
5. Hydrocortisone hemisuccinate enemas
6. For severe attack
   a. Parenteral feeding
   b. ACTH or systemic steroids

SURGICAL THERAPY

Indications
1. Lack of response to medical therapy
2. Perforation
3. Massive hemorrhage
4. Toxic megacolon unresponsive to 48 hours of medical therapy. Use Turnbull "blow-hole" if not perforated
5. Carcinoma
6. Some extracolonic manifestations (such as recurrent polyarthritis)

Techniques
1. Total proctocolectomy with permanent ileostomy
2. Rectal preservation debated

Complications
1. Impotence in 10 to 15 percent of men
2. Many operative complications possible

PROGNOSIS

1. Colectomy eventually required in 15 percent of cases
2. Operative mortality rate: 3 percent elective, 5 to 10 percent emergency

CROHN'S DISEASE

PATHOLOGY

1. Transmural process
2. Thickened bowel with thick exudate
3. Mesenteric fat growing over serosa

4. Adhesions
5. Lymph node masses
6. Thickened mesentery
7. "Skip" pattern

ETIOLOGY (unknown)

1. "Slow" virus (?)
2. *Yersinia enterocolitica*—found in *acute* terminal ileitis

PATTERNS OF INVOLVEMENT

1. Small bowel (usually terminal ileum)—60 percent
2. Large bowel—17 percent
3. Both small and large bowel—17 percent
4. Anorectal—rare

INCIDENCE

1. Mainly young adults (especially terminal ileum)
2. Another peak at 70 years (especially rectosigmoid)

CLINICAL FINDINGS (often of years' duration)

1. Diarrhea
2. Weight loss, anorexia, anemia
3. Abdominal pain, low-grade fever, abdominal mass
4. Polyarthritis and spondylitis (especially in colonic form)
5. Uveitis, pyoderma gangrenosa
6. Complications (listed under "Surgical Therapy")

DIAGNOSIS

Laboratory Results
1. Low serum albumin, anemia
2. Abnormal D-xylose absorption
3. High serum lysozyme level

Small Bowel Barium Series or Barium Enema (See Fig. 18-4)
1. "String sign" = thickened bowel wall and stricture
2. Cobblestone formation
3. Deep transverse fissures, longitudinal ulceration
4. Fistula, abscess
5. "Skip" lesions

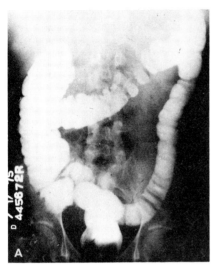

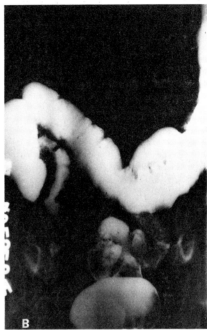

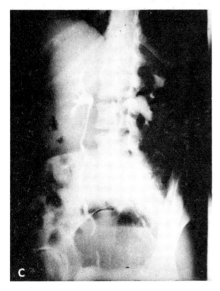

Figure 18-4 Normal barium enema (A) and one showing thickened bowel wall and narrowing in terminal ileum characteristic of Crohn's disease (B). Left hydroureter due to retroperitoneal inflammation in severe Crohn's disease is shown on the intravenous pyelogram (C).

COLONIC CROHN'S DISEASE: DIFFERENTIATION FROM ULCERATIVE COLITIS

	Crohn's colitis (transmural)	Ulcerative colitis (mucosal)
Pattern of involvement	"Skip" lesions	Uniformly granular mucosa
Rectal bleeding		More common
Perianal fistulas	More common	
Toxic dilatation		More common
Recurrence	More common	
X-ray	Segmental, strictures, fistulas	Shortening of colon, pseudopolyposis, loss of haustral markings
Carcinoma	Seldom	More frequent

MEDICAL THERAPY (debated)

1. Bed rest, diet
   a. Low residue diet
   b. Elemental diet
   c. Hyperalimentation
      i. Nutritional adjunct to other therapy
      ii. In preparation for surgery
2. Medications
   a. Antispasmodics
   b. Azulfidine (sulfasalazine)—0.5 g po qid
   c. Prednisone—initially 20 to 30 mg daily
   d. Azathioprine
   e. ACTH
   f. Metronidazole (Flagyl)—active against anaerobes

SURGICAL THERAPY

Indications
1. Unresponsiveness to medical therapy
2. Complications
   a. Internal or perianal fistulas
   b. Abscesses
   c. Free perforation (rare)
   d. Intestinal obstruction
   e. Bleeding (rare)
   f. Obstructive uropathy
3. Carcinoma—rare, but has poor prognosis due to difficulty of diagnosis

Procedures (many)
1. En-bloc resection of symptomatic areas, *not* including proximal skip areas
2. Drainage alone—for very sick patients with abscess
3. Defunction diseased bowel
   a. Diverting ileostomy

   b. Ileotransverse colostomy
      i. High incidence of fistula formation
      ii. May lead to asymptomatic carcinoma
      iii. Indicated in elderly patient with obstruction due to fibrosis
4. No procedure or appendectomy alone
   a. If operating for suspected appendicitis, and unsuspected Crohn's disease discovered
   b. Appendectomy in general recommended only if cecum *not* involved
   c. These patients usually will *not* require further surgery
5. Other procedures
   a. Ureterolysis—for obstructive uropathy
   b. Colectomy—for colonic Crohn's disease
   c. Bilroth II or gastroenterostomy—for duodenal Crohn's disease

Complications
1. Mortality—3 percent at first procedure, increases subsequently
2. Recurrence rate—reported at 30 to 90 percent—usually in bowel *proximal* to anastomosis, least with primary resection

HEMORRHOIDS

ANATOMY (See Fig. 18-5)

Muscle
1. Internal sphincter (bulbous thickening of colonic circular muscle coat)
2. External sphincter (circular muscle) in three portions
   a. Superficial
   b. Subcutaneous
   c. Deep
3. Levator ani
4. To preserve continence, must leave at least one portion of external sphincter or levator intact

Venous Drainage
1. Above dentate line (internal hemorrhoids): superior hemorrhoidal vein to inferior mesenteric vein to portal system
2. Below dentate line (external hemorrhoids): inferior and middle hemorrhoidal veins to hypogastric vein to vena cava

Usual Locations of Internal Hemorrhoids
1. (R) anterior
2. (R) posterior
3. (L) lateral

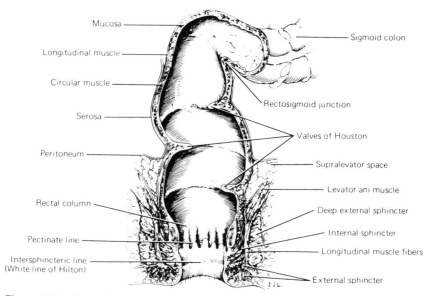

Figure 18-5   Normal anatomy of rectum and anal canal. *(From Dunphy JE and Way LW (eds):* Current Surgical Diagnosis and Treatment, *3rd Edt. Lange, 1977, p 654, with permission.)*

ETIOLOGY

1. Infected material → anal crypt → ducts → glands → lymphatics → vein walls
2. Hereditary disposition
3. Straining at stool
4. Portal hypertension (?)
5. Pregnancy

TREATMENT

1. R/O associated pathology (proctoscopy, BE)
2. If thrombosed—evacuate clot
3. If acutely inflamed—medical therapy
4. If not acutely inflamed but symptomatic—hemorrhoidectomy

Techniques
1. Submucosal technique
   a. Tedious dissection of veins with ligation
   b. Leave wound open
   c. Increased incidence of bleeding
2. Closed technique
   a. Excise triangular wedge of skin + mucosa + hemorrhoids

  b. Suture closed completely
  c. Abscess rate: only 0.2 percent
  d. Minimal bleeding
3. Rubberband ligation
  a. Limited to uncomplicated *internal* hemorrhoids
  b. Problem: no specimen to pathology
4. Wide anal dilatation alone: assumes that stricture is primary pathology

Complications

1. Bleeding
2. Infection
3. Stricture: prevent with four-finger dilatation intraoperatively, bulky stools, preservation of mucosa
4. Incidental carcinoma in excised tissue
  a. Incidence: 1.9 percent
  b. Treatment: wider local excision, follow-up observation

ANAL FISSURE

PATHOLOGY

1. Denuded epithelium usually in posterior midline → edema and hypertrophy of papille → lymphatic obstruction → fibrosis of skin at anal verge ("Sentinel pile")

ETIOLOGY

1. Irritant stools
2. Muscular spasm
3. Trauma

CLINICAL FINDINGS

1. Severely painful defecation
2. Blood on paper

DIAGNOSIS

1. Observation of sentinel pile
2. Pain and spasm on digital exam
3. *Defer* sigmoidoscopy until acute episode resolves

MEDICAL THERAPY

1. Stool softener, sitz baths, topical ointments (Mantadil cream)

SURGICAL THERAPY

1. Indicated for intolerable pain or chronicity
2. Method is
   a. Excise sentinel pile (promotes drainage), and
   b. Lateral internal sphincterotomy
   c. Local anesthesia may be used

SELECTED BIBLIOGRAPHY

Beart RW Jr, McIlrath DC, Kelly KA, et al.: Surgical management of inflammatory bowel disease. Curr Probl Surg 17(10): October 1980
Goligher JC, et al.: Surgery of the Anus, Rectum and Colon, 4th Edt. London, Bailliere Tindall, 1980
Sugerbaker PH: Carcinoma of the colon—prognosis and operative choice. Curr Probl Surg 18(12): December 1981

QUESTIONS

DIRECTIONS: Each of the questions or incomplete statements below is followed by five suggested answers or completions. Select the *one* that is *best* in each case.

1. The treatment of choice for a 20-year-old female with familial polyposis is:
   A. Biannual sigmoidoscopy
   B. Biannual sigmoidoscopy and barium enema
   C. Fulguration of all polyps
   D. Subtotal colectomy
   E. No specific treatment is necessary
2. A 70-year-old female states that she has noted spots of red blood on otherwise normal brown stool. The most likely etiology is:
   A. Cancer of the colon
   B. Cancer of the rectum
   C. Squamous cell cancer of the anus
   D. Diverticulosis
   E. Hemorrhoids
3. A 60-year-old man presents with a history of intermittent constipation and recurrent left lower quadrant abdominal pain. On physical examination he has mild tenderness and minimal rebound tenderness in his left lower

quadrant. Bowel sounds are normal. Rectal examination is negative. Stool hematest is negative. Proctoscopy is negative to 15 cm, where further progression of the proctoscope is impossible. In view of these findings, the most likely diagnosis is:

A. Crohn's disease
B. Cancer of the colon
C. Diverticulitis
D. Sigmoid volvulus
E. Ruptured appendicitis

4. An adenocarcinoma found on rectal examination at 3 cm from the anal verge is best treated by:

A. Left hemicolectomy
B. Total proctocolectomy
C. Abdominoperineal resection
D. Anterior resection of the colon
E. Radiotherapy and chemotherapy only

5. Of the following, the most common malignancy to first present as an abdominal mass is:

A. Uterine cancer
B. Ovarian cancer
C. Cancer of the right colon
D. Cancer of the left colon
E. Cancer of the stomach

6. Which of the following colonic lesions is most likely to be accompanied by a malignancy?

A. Villous adenoma
B. Hamartoma
C. Adenomatous polyp
D. Crohn's disease
E. Juvenile polyps

7. Watery diarrhea and hypokalemia are typically associated with which of the following lesions of the colon and rectum?

A. Gardner's syndrome
B. Peutz-Jeghers syndrome
C. Villous adenoma
D. Juvenile polyps
E. Pseudopolyposis

8. A permanent colostomy would most likely be required in the surgical treatment of which of the following?

A. Crohn's disease of the colon
B. Ulcerative colitis
C. Peutz-Jeghers syndrome
D. Cancer of the rectum discovered on digital examination
E. Large, fungating mass found at 25 centimeters on sigmoidoscopy

9. Bright red blood streaking of stool associated with excruciating pain on defecation suggests:

A. Rectal cancer

B. Condylomata accuminata
C. Anal fissure
D. Anal fistula
E. Internal hemorrhoids

10. Prevention of postoperative pseudomembranous enterocolitis requires:
    A. Use of preoperative stool softeners
    B. Antibiotic bowel preparation
    C. Avoidance of nonabsorbable colonic sutures
    D. Adequate resection margins
    E. Avoidance of unnecessary antibiotics

11. Obstruction of which of the following is *least* likely to cause early vomiting?
    A. Gastric outlet
    B. High small bowel
    C. Large bowel
    D. Ureter
    E. Appendix

12. A chronically low-fiber diet has been suspected in the pathogenesis of each of the following *except:*
    A. Sigmoid volvulus
    B. Hemorrhoids
    C. Cancer of the colon
    D. Diverticular disease of the colon
    E. Appendicitis

ANSWERS

1. **D** Familial polyposis is inherited as an autosomal dominant and results in the occurrence of a blanket of adenomatous polyps throughout the colon. It has a high tendency toward malignancy, reaching 100 percent by age 40, and is treated by subtotal colectomy and ileoproctostomy; that is, removing the colon but leaving the rectum in place. The rectum can then be observed by routine proctoscopies and new polyps fulgurated. When familial polyposis occurs with osteomas and sebaceous cysts it is called Gardner's Syndrome.

2. **E** This is a classic presentation for hemorrhoids, but rectal examination and sigmoidoscopy must be performed to rule out the possibility of cancer and to confirm the existence of hemorrhoids.

3. **C** This is a typical case of sigmoid diverticulitis with a small abscess in the sigmoid mesentery. Inflammatory changes due to the underlying disease lead to rigidity of the sigmoid mesentery and make passage of the proctoscope beyond 15 cm difficult. Although colon cancer cannot be ruled out based on the findings, the fact that the stool is Hematest-negative would make this diagnosis less likely. Sigmoid volvulus would present with severe pain, abdominal distention, no stool in the rectum, and hyperactive, high-pitched bowel sounds.

4. **C** Lesions below 7 cm must be removed by abdominoperineal resection (Miles procedure), which results in permanent colostomy. Anterior resection (colon resection with anastomosis below the peritoneal reflection) is appropriate for higher rectal lesions. In selected, high-risk patients, low-lying lesions can be treated with fulguration.

5. **C** Cancer of the left colon commonly obstructs due to the solid nature of the fecal material at this point. Cancers of the right colon may grow to a large size before they produce obstruction and therefore often present with a palpable mass as their earliest finding.

6. **A** Villous adenomas of the colon are notoriously premalignant. They are also associated with diarrhea and hypokalemia.

7. **C** Villous adenoma, again.

8. **D** Abdominoperineal resection (Miles procedure) is used for resectable cancers of the rectum within 7 centimeters of the anal verge. It requires a permanent (end) colostomy. Lesions higher than this may be treated with anterior resection, in which the anastomosis is performed below the peritoneal reflection and, if tenuous, may require a temporary protective colostomy, but not a permanent colostomy. Ulcerative colitis may or may not be treated with proctocolectomy. If it is, the end result is a permanent ileostomy, not colostomy.

9. **C** This is a typical picture of an acute fissure-in-ano, a tear in the mucosa. Treatment is sitz baths, local ointments, stool softeners. Sphincterotomy is reserved for chronic fissures.

10. **E** Pseudomembranous enterocolitis is an uncommon complication following the overuse of antibiotics. Elimination of normal colonic flora leads to overgrowth of resistant staphylococci and clostridia with destruction of mucosa. This causes diarrhea, abdominal distention, hypotension, and shock. Prevention entails avoidance of prolonged courses of preoperative antiobitc therapy. Treatment is NG suction, IV fluids, and appropriate antibiotics directed against the offending organism.

11. **C** Obstruction of the lumen of the appendix initially causes periumbilical pain and then reflex vomiting. Gastric outlet obstruction and high small bowel obstruction cause early vomiting due to gastric distention. Ureteral obstruction causes early and severe reflex vomiting. Large bowel obstruction causes little vomiting, especially if the ileocecal valve is competent, thereby preventing reflux of material into the small bowel.

12. **A** A diet which is chronically low in fiber, by producing inappropriate muscular segmentation of the colon, tends to lead to diverticulitis and possible appendicitis. Chronically increased intraabdominal pressure may cause hemorrhoids and even varicose veins. An increased concentration of carcinogens resulting from little bulk in the colon may lead to colon cancer. On the other hand, African tribes eating nothing but fiber tend to have a very high incidence of sigmoid volvulus.

19. Peripheral Arteries

NORMAL ARTERIAL WALL

1. Intima = endothelium + connective tissue in subendothelial layer
2. Internal elastic membrane
3. Media
   a. Muscle fibers—greatest in medium-sized vessels
   b. Elastic tissue—greatest in large-sized vessels
4. External elastic membrane
5. Adventitia
   a. Best developed in medium-sized arteries
   b. Carries vasa vasorum (nutrient vessels)

STAGES OF ATHEROSCLEROTIC PROCESS (See Fig. 19-1)

1. Asymptomatic: fatty streaks, fibrous plaques
2. Potentially symptomatic: calcification, hemorrhage, ulceration, thrombosis
3. Ischemic: occlusive thrombosis with end-organ ischemia

ASSOCIATED FACTORS

1. Diet—high in saturated fat and cholesterol
2. Hyperlipidemia
   a. Primary—genetic defect (See below)
   b. Secondary—due to: hypothyroidism, nephrotic syndrome, diabetes mellitus, biliary obstruction
3. Hypertension
4. Diabetes mellitus
5. Hyperuricemia and gout
6. Cigarette smoking
7. EKG abnormalities

BIOCHEMISTRY OF HYPERLIPIDEMIA

1. Lipids insoluble in blood, hence bound to proteins
2. Classified based on ultracentrifugation
   a. Low-density lipoproteins (beta)

STAGE I ASYMPTOMATIC	STAGE II SYMPTOMATIC	STAGE III COMPLICATIONS

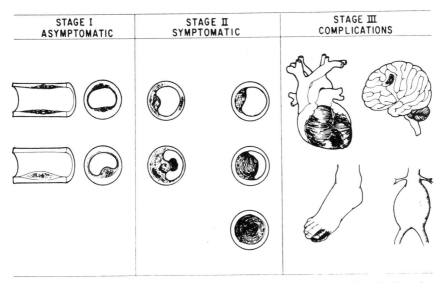

Figure 19-1 The natural history of arteriosclerosis. *(From Haimovici H (ed):* Vascular Surgery. Principles and Techniques. *McGraw-Hill, 1976, p 214, with permission.)*

b. Very low density lipoproteins (prebeta)
c. High density lipoproteins (alpha) increase of HDL may actually *decrease* risk of heart attack
d. Chylomicrons = exogenous triglycerides and proteins via intestinal lymphatics to plasma

PATHOGENESIS (uncertain)

1. Lipid metabolism—increased blood lipoproteins settle in avascular connective tissue (intima)
2. Thrombogenic theory—fibrin deposits lead to fibrous thickenings
3. Pressure-flow factors—turbulence causes plaque formation
4. Role of arterial wall—endogenous cholesterol synthesis

DIAGNOSIS

Physical Examination
1. Pulses, bruits, thrills, diminished pulses after exercise, color of extremity after exercise, aneurysm, neurologic examination

Noninvasive Procedures
1. *Doppler ultrasonic flow detector*
   a. Can measure systolic blood pressure in extremities (radial, brachial, popliteal, dorsalis pedis, posterior tibial arteries)

    b. Ankle/arm pressure ratio normally at least 1.0
2. *Plethysmography*—estimates blood flow to extremity in terms of changing circumference with heart beats, or after proximal venous occlusion
3. *Sonography*
    a. For suspected abdominal aortic aneurysm
    b. For evaluation of superficial vessels (requires high resolution equipment): carotid, femoral
4. *Digital subtraction angiography (DSA)* = computer-enhanced arteriogram obtained from intravenous dye injection; *relatively* noninvasive outpatient procedure

Arteriography
1. *Methods*
    a. Direct puncture: translumbar aortogram, carotid puncture, femoral puncture
    b. Transfemoral or transaxillary catheter: preferred method
2. Multiple views (oblique, lateral, PA) may be necessary if suspected plaque is not easily visualized
3. Information obtained: location of disease, nature of disease, distal vasculature ("runoff")
4. Complications: hematoma, dislodgement of plaque, renal failure due to dye (make certain patient is well hydrated), allergic reactions

Intraoperative Studies
1. Doppler flow or pressure measurements
2. Electromagnetic flow measurement
3. Intraoperative arteriography

TREATMENT

Medical
1. Eliminate risk factors: smoking, hypertension, uncontrolled diabetes, hyperlipidemia, obesity
2. Exercise: walk with claudication to increase collateral flow
3. Vasodilators, anticoagulants (efficacy debated)

▶ DECISION MAKING IN LOWER EXTREMITY VASCULAR DISEASE

Decisions concerning operative management of lower extremity vascular disease are often difficult. They may be based to some extent on the following rough approximations:
1. 1 percent—Mortality rate of major vascular bypass; rate of major complications of transfemoral angiography
2. 10 percent—Frequency of gangrene within 10 years after onset of claudication (unoperated)

3. 20 percent—Frequency of non-healing of below-knee (B-K) amputation requiring above-knee (A-K) amputation
4. 30 percent—5-year survival after A-K or B-K amputation
5. 40 percent—5-year patency of axillofemoral bypass
6. 50 percent—Frequency of contralateral amputation required within 1-year of A-K
7. 60 percent—Overall improvement rate with lumbar sympathectomy (varies substantially with indication)
8. 70 percent—5-year patency rate of femorotibial bypass
9. 80 percent—5-year patency of femoropopliteal bypass
10. 90 percent—5-year patency rate of aortofemoral bypass

Surgical

1. *Endarterectomy:* removal of intima and plaque; limited to short-segment lesions
2. *Bypass:* requires good "runoff" to assure graft patency
   a. Materials: autogenous vein (usually saphenous)—highest patency rates, expanded polytetrafluorethylene, Dacron, bovine heterograft
   b. Problems: graft occlusion, infection potentiated by foreign body
3. *Percutaneous transluminal angioplasty*
   a. Method: balloon dilatation under fluoroscopic control
   b. Requires: isolated, hemodynamically-significant, short-segment lesion
   c. Contraindicated: if atheroembolism suspected; thrombosis; long-segment lesion
   d. Complications: thrombosis, embolization, vessel rupture, recurrence (common)

ARTERIAL EMBOLISM

SOURCE

1. Heart (90 percent)
   a. Atherosclerotic heart disease
      i. Myocardial infarction
      ii. Left ventricular mural thrombi over infarct
      iii. May embolize *before* MI manifests clinically ("silent MI")
   b. Rheumatic valvular disease: left atrial thrombi in mitral stenosis
   c. Atrial fibrillation (60 to 70 percent)
   d. Bacterial endocarditis (rare)
   e. Atrial myxoma (rare): diagnosis can be made by pathologic examination of embolus.
2. Distal aorta—atheroembolism
3. Paradoxical emboli—venous through right-to-left intracardiac shunt

Location (usually at bifurcations)	Percent
Subclavian/axillary	4.5
Brachial	9.1
Radial/ulnar	2.4
Aortic bifurcation	9.1
Common iliac	13.6
External iliac	3.0
Femoral	34.0
Profunda femoris	—
Popliteal	14.2
Anterior tibial	2.8
Posterior tibial	2.8
Peroneal	—
Visceral arteries	5–10

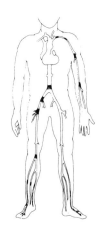

Figure 19-2 Location of peripheral arterial emboli.

DIAGNOSIS

▶ **Findings ("The five Ps")**
1. Paresthesias
2. Pain
3. Pulselessness
4. Pallor
5. Paralysis

Note: stiff calf suggests necrosis

Other
1. Plethysmography; Doppler assessment
2. Arteriography: only if extent of thrombus is not certain clinically or if atheroembolism suspected. Do *not* delay embolectomy for arteriography

TREATMENT

1. Immediate heparinization
2. Early balloon embolectomy (optimal time less than 12 hours)
3. Even late embolectomy is useful if limb appears salvageable
4. Untreated → gangrene in 50 percent

TECHNIQUE (See Fig. 19-3)

1. Usually transfemoral under local anesthesia for lower limb embolus at any site
2. May on occasion require exposure of popliteal artery
3. For aortic bifurcation ("saddle") embolus, use bifemoral route

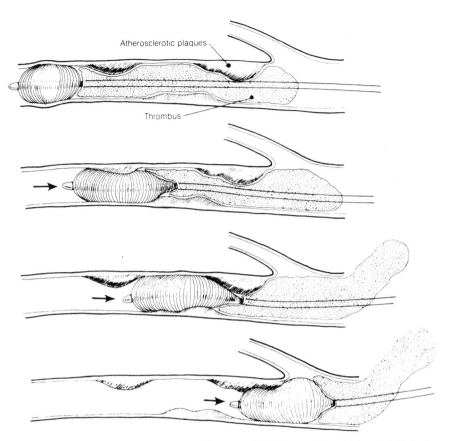

Figure 19-3 Technique of balloon catheter embolectomy. *(From Haimovici H (ed): Vascular Surgery. Principles and Techniques. McGraw-Hill, 1976, p 285, with permission.)*

OUTCOME OF EMBOLECTOMY DEPENDS UPON

1. Undamaged intima
2. Nonadherence of embolus and secondary thrombus to intima
3. Patent distal tree prior to embolism
4. Pretreatment with anticoagulants

COMPLICATIONS

1. Venous thrombosis
2. Venous embolism (pulmonary)
3. Muscle ischemia (fasciotomy if tense edema occurs)

4. Myopathic-nephrotic-metabolic syndrome
  a. Clinical findings
     i. Excruciating pain
     ii. Pronounced ischemia
     iii. Rigidity of limb (rigor mortis)
     iv. Massive edema
  b. Metabolic derangements after embolectomy
     i. Metabolic (lactic) acidosis
     ii. Low Po_2
     iii. Hyperkalemia
     iv. Increased CPK, LDH, and SGOT
  c. Therapy
     i. Sodium bicarbonate
     ii. Dialysis
     iii. *Amputation*
5. Catheter-related complications
  a. Arterial rupture
  b. Arterial perforation
  c. Intimal dissection
  d. Breakage of catheter with embolization of rubber
  e. Avulsion of atherosclerotic plaques
  f. Impaction of thrombus distally
  g. Shifting of thrombus to another vessel
  h. Arteriovenous fistula
6. Death
  a. Usually due to preexistent heart disease
  b. 5-year survival rate is about 45 percent overall

AORTOILIAC OCCLUSIVE DISEASE

COLLATERAL CIRCULATION

1. Superior mesenteric artery →
   Middle colic artery →
   Marginal artery of mesentery (Drummond) →
   Inferior mesenteric artery →
   Superior hemorrhoidal artery →
   Pelvic vessels →
   Illiac artery
2. Winslow's system:
   Intercostals, internal mammary, inferior epigastric

CLINICAL FINDINGS

1. Claudication: hip claudication is due to occlusion of internal iliacs
2. Rest pain
3. Gangrene
4. LeRiche syndrome = sexual impotence + claudication due to aortoiliac bifurcation disease (See Fig. 19-4)

INDICATIONS FOR OPERATION

1. Disabling claudication unresponsive to medical therapy
2. Ischemic rest pain (originates in toes or metatarsal heads and is relieved by dependency)
3. Threatened limb loss (claudication alone does not threaten limb loss)
4. Sudden occlusion due to embolism from heart, pathologic embolism from venous side through septal defect, atheroembolism from proximal plaque, or thrombosis (commonly due to hypotension)
5. Arteriogram shows lesions that might lead to sudden occlusion with acute ischemia

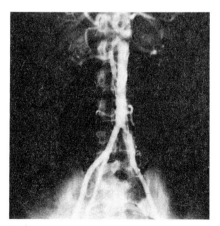 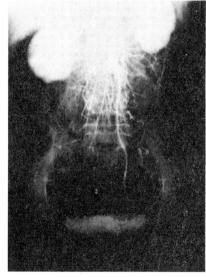

Figure 19-4 Transfemoral aortogram showing segmental occlusion of the left common iliac artery (left); one showing total occlusion of the infrarenal abdominal aorta- runoff via renal arteries keeps aorta open at that level (right).

OPERATION

1. Aortoiliac thromboendarterectomy: for limited disease or recurrent atheroembolism
2. Aortoiliac or aortofemoral bypass: indicated for occlusion over 6 to 8 cm in length, severe calcification or small caliber vessels
3. Femorofemoral bypass: for unilateral iliac occlusion especially in poor-risk patients since local anesthesia may be used (See Fig. 19-5)
4. Axillofemoral bypass: also using local anesthesia in poor-risk patients
5. Percutaneous transluminal angioplasty: for high grade, non-embolizing, iliac stenosis

DISEASE PROGRESSION POSTOPERATIVELY

1. Inversely proportional to blood flow through involved vessel: hence, iliac *donor* site of femorofemoral bypass has good prognosis

COMPLICATIONS OF OPERATION

Intraoperative
1. Bleeding from
   a. Lumbar veins

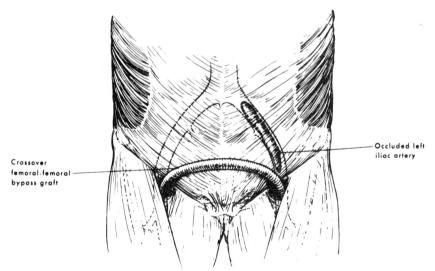

Figure 19-5 Use of the femorofemoral crossover graft for unilateral iliac artery occlusion. *(From Haimovici H (ed):* Vascular Surgery. Principles and Techniques. *McGraw-Hill, 1976, p 586, with permission.)*

b. Anomalous renal veins

c. Anomalous vena cava

2. Left renal vein may be safely divided to increase exposure
3. Renal ischemia due to injury to anomalous renal artery, or horseshoe kidney
4. Intestinal ischemia due to ligation of IMA if SMA occluded

Postoperative

1. Renal failure: prevent with intraoperative furosemide (Lasix)
2. Arterial occlusion: prevent with adequate heparinization
3. Hemorrhage: prevent by preclotting graft, and may reverse heparin with Protamine
4. Anterior spinal syndrome (paraplegia)
5. Infected graft: treatment is removal and extraanatomic bypass (See Fig. 19-6)
6. Renal artery embolus
7. Decubitus ulcers—in part, results from ischemia during aortic occlusion
8. Pseudoaneurysm: rare now that synthetic suture material is used routinely
9. Aortoenteric fistula: usually duodenum. Prevent by carefully closing retroperitoneum or omental interposition
10. Prolonged ileus

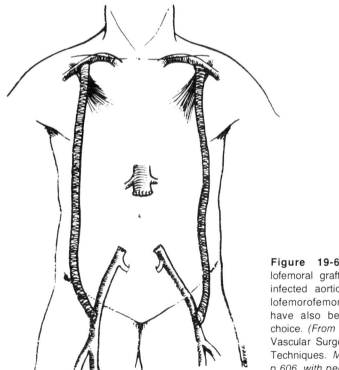

Figure 19-6 Bilateral axillofemoral graft after removal of infected aortic prosthesis. Axillofemorofemoral bypass would have also been a satisfactory choice. *(From Haimovici H (ed):* Vascular Surgery. Principles and Techniques. *McGraw-Hill, 1976, p 606, with permission.)*

11. Numerous systemic complications due to associated diseases
12. Death: 2.5 to 5 percent in elective cases

Reasons for Occlusion of Graft
1. Poor runoff (disease distal to anastomosis)
2. Technical error
3. Hypotensive episode
4. Thrombogenic graft material

FEMOROPOPLITEAL OCCLUSIVE DISEASE

COLLATERAL CIRCULATION

1. Occlusion of common femoral: iliac arteries → iliolumbar, superior gluteal, inferior gluteal, obturator, deep iliac circumflex → profunda femoris branches
2. Occlusion of superficial femoral (See Fig. 19-7): profunda femoris branches (especially descending branch of lateral circumflex and rectus femoral collateral) → genicular network
3. Occlusion of popliteal: genicular network → recurrent tibial arteries
4. Occlusion of leg arteries: many other small vessels

OPERATION

1. Femoropopliteal bypass using
   a. Saphenous vein (reversed)—preferred
   b. Saphenous vein (nonreversed, in situ)
      i. Advantages: maximal blood velocity in critical distal area, intact vasa vasorum, avoids twisting of graft
      ii. Disadvantages: must destroy valves, must ligate perforating tributaries to avoid A-V fistulas
   c. Expanded polytetraflorethylene (PTFE)
2. Endarterectomy
   a. Especially used in local area of implantation of graft
   b. Must avoid distal intimal flap
3. Profundaplasty: early branching usually keeps profunda open even with advanced disease of superficial femoral
   a. By endarterectomy with patch graft
   b. Quick procedure, local anesthesia possible
   c. Use if poor runoff makes femoropopliteal bypass impossible

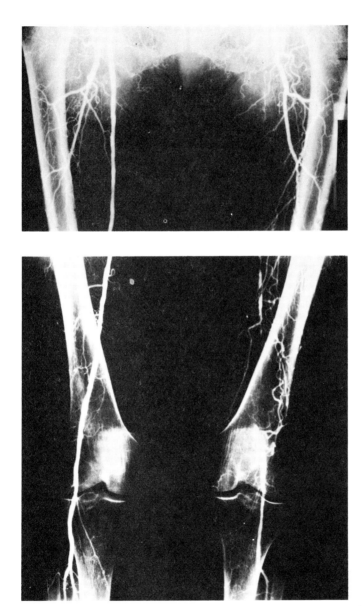

Figure 19-7 Femoropopliteal occlusive disease. Arteriogram showing occlusion of the left superficial femoral artery with good distal runoff from profunda collaterals. This patient did well after femoropopliteal bypass. (Right femoral is normal).

COMPLICATIONS OF OPERATION

1. Occlusion of graft
   a. Saphenous graft has highest patency rate
   b. Morbidity and limb loss is higher in patients with unsuccessful bypass graft than in those not operated for claudication
   c. Patency rates vary—about 40 percent overall for patients surviving 10 years
2. Mortality
   a. Related to associated diseases
   b. Varies, but about 75 percent mortality at 10 years

ABDOMINAL AORTIC ANEURYSM

ETIOLOGY

1. Atherosclerosis
2. Mycotic (infection): subacute bacterial endocarditis, syphilitic
3. Traumatic: may be true or false aneurysm

INCIDENCE

1. Age—seventh decade average
2. Sex—M:F = 9:1

LOCATION

1. Starts just below renals
2. Suprarenal—rare except as part of thoracoabdominal aneurysm

DIAGNOSIS

1. Palpation: must differentiate from tortuous (S-shaped) aorta
2. Plain x-ray: calcific outline visible in one-half of cases (See Fig. 19-8)
3. Echography: diagnostic in almost 100 percent of cases
4. Aortography
   a. Diagnostic value limited because of laminated thrombus preventing visualization
   b. Sometimes important in determining associated vascular occlusive diseases

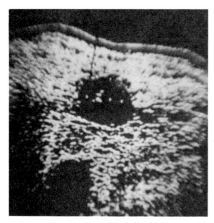 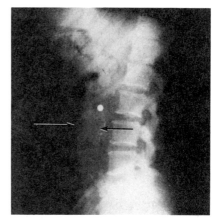

Figure 19-8 Lateral abdominal x-ray showing the calcific outline of an abdominal aortic aneurysm (right), sonogram confirming infrarenal aortic aneurysm (left).

OTHER STUDIES

1. Intravenous pyelography—to rule out horseshoe kidney
2. Evaluate heart and cerebral circulation
2. If fever/leukocytosis or vertebral erosion, rule out infected aneurysm with blood cultures (most often *Staphylococcus* or *Salmonella*)

THERAPY

1. Aneurysmectomy with
   a. Aortoiliac bypass (usually), or
   b. Aortofemoral bypass (if severe atherosclerosis involving iliacs), or
   c. Aortic tube graft (for small aneurysm not involving bifurcation)
2. If mycotic aneurysm
   a. Excise, and use
   b. Extraanatomic bypass (axillofemoral or thoracoiliac)

OPERATIVE COMPLICATIONS

1. Peripheral embolization
2. Venous laceration
3. Ischemia of rectosigmoid
   a. *Treatment:* reimplantation of inferior mesenteric artery and exteriorization of bowel
4. Paraplegia (due to spinal cord ischemia)
5. "Declamping phenomenon"
   a. Due to release of toxic metabolites

b. Manifested by acidosis, hypotension, hypoxemia
c. May lead to renal failure
6. Sexual disturbances

COINCIDENTAL MALIGNANCY

Incidence
1. 4 percent of cases
2. Usually colorectal, lung, or genitourinary tract

Treatment
1. If aneurysm is symptomatic or impending rupture, treat aneurysm first
2. If malignancy bleeding, perforated, or obstructed, treat malignancy first
3. Otherwise, treat aneurysm if very large, or malignancy if aneurysm is small

RUPTURED ANEURYSM

Location
1. Usually occurs on left posterior wall
2. 2 to 5 cm below renals
3. Usually hematoma is purely retroperitoneal

Diagnosis
1. *Pain* (abdominal, back, or left flank with radiation to groin)
2. Ecchymosis of flanks or perineum
3. Femoral neuropathy (rare)
4. Hemorrhagic shock
5. Oliguria

Therapy
1. Immediate surgery
2. DO NOT WAIT for x-ray confirmation!

Prognosis
1. Depends on extent of hematoma
2. Grave if intraperitoneal rupture

Factors Contributing to Lower Mortality in Emergency Aneurysmectomy
1. Adequate intravenous therapy (prevents renal failure); e.g.:

Operative	3 to 4 liter D_5RL
	½ liter D_5W
	blood as lost
First day	1 liter D_5RL
	2½ liter D_5W

Second day   ½ liter D$_5$RL
                                      2 liter D$_5$W
2. Rapid aortic cross-clamping just subdiaphragmatic, or via left lateral thoracotomy
3. Use of nonporous (*woven*) graft: preclotted *knitted* grafts will bleed profusely, since these patients have lost much of their clotting ability or are heparinized preoperatively
4. Intraoperative autotransfusion
5. Immediate and rapid operation: anesthetize after prep and drape

Rare Sites of Rupture
1. Into inferior vena cava
   a. High-output cardiac failure
   b. Hepatomegaly
   c. Engorged veins of lower extremities
   d. Machinery-like bruit
2. Into left renal vein
3. Aortoenteric fistula (usually duodenal)
   a. Present with GI bleeding and back pain
   b. Problem is graft in face of retroperitoneal sepsis

LUMBAR SYMPATHECTOMY

ANATOMY/PHYSIOLOGY (See Fig. 19-9)

1. Remove L2 to L4 ganglia
2. Increases skin blood flow
3. Does not increase muscle blood flow (may decrease)

INDICATIONS (debated)

1. Disease not amenable to direct arterial reconstruction on the basis of arteriography, and
2. Gangrene involving less than distal one-half of foot (this may allow transmetatarsal instead of B-K amputation)
3. Ulcerative ischemic lesions
4. Rest pain
5. Adjunct to reconstructive procedures
6. Raynaud's phenomenon
7. Frostbite, hyperhidrosis, or causalgia
8. Buerger's disease (thromboangiitis obliterans): patient *must* stop smoking

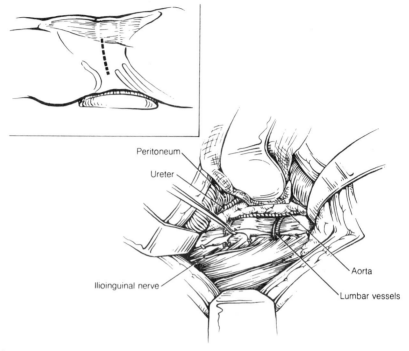

Figure 19-9 Anatomical relationships in left lumbar sympathectomy. *(From Haimovici H (ed): Vascular Surgery. Principles and Techniques. McGraw-Hill, 1976, p 783, with permission.)*

CONTRAINDICATIONS

1. Gangrene of more than one-half of foot or of proximal foot
2. Intermittent claudication alone
3. Not to be used as a substitute for arterial reconstructive surgery

COMPLICATIONS

1. Retrograde ejaculation (results from bilateral removal of L1)
2. Ileus
3. Neuralgia (prevent by clipping ends of divided chain)

AUTOSYMPATHECTOMY

1. Thought to result from peripheral neuropathy in diabetics
2. This probably does *not* occur

EFFECTIVENESS

1. About 60 percent overall improvement
2. Dependent on indication

AMPUTATION

SELECTION OF SITE

1. "The longer, the better"
2. Feasibility of rehabilitation
   a. Proximal amputation for bedridden patient
   b. Amputate above level of contracture
3. Blood supply judged by
   a. Pulses
   b. Bleeding from incision
   c. Histamine wheal
4. Knee joint is preserved if possible

LEVELS (See Fig. 19-10)

1. Toe, ray, transmetatarsal, Syme (not recommended for vascular disease because long heel flap may become ischemic), B-K, knee disarticulation, A-K, hip disarticulation

TECHNIQUE

1. Standard
2. Osteomyoplastic and myodesis
   a. Improved function
   b. Allows immediate postsurgical prosthesis
3. Open ("guillotine") (See Fig. 19-11)
   a. Drainage procedure in toxic patients
   b. Requires later revision
4. Paradoxical
   a. Freezing of extremity as temporary measure
   b. Use tourniquet above frozen area
   c. Only in gravely ill patients

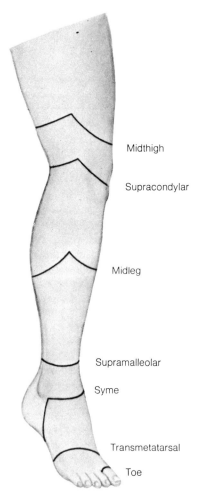

Midthigh

Supracondylar

Midleg

Supramalleolar

Syme

Transmetatarsal

Toe

Figure 19-10 Levels of amputation for ischemic gangrene. *(From Haimovici H (ed):* Vascular Surgery. Principles and Techniques. *McGraw-Hill, 1976, p 896, with permission.)*

REQUIREMENTS FOR B-K OVER A-K

1. Patient able to walk
2. Skin satisfactory at B-K level (long posterior flap)
3. Femoral pulse intact
4. Patent profunda femoris
5. Intact knee joint

REHABILITATION

1. Immediate postoperative prosthesis and rigid plaster dressing are debated—may impair healing of stump

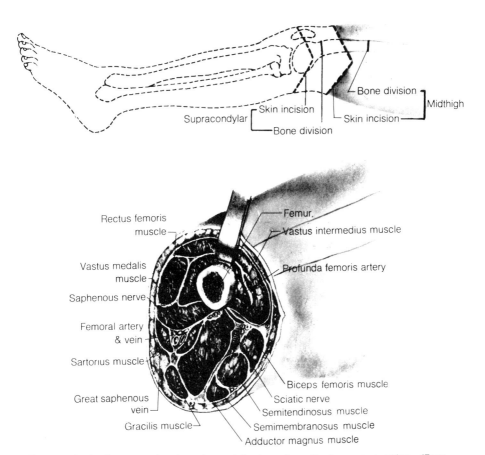

Figure 19-11 Cross sectional anatomy following above-the-knee amputation. *(From Haimovici H (ed): Vascular Surgery. Principles and Techniques. McGraw-Hill, 1976, p 918, with permission.)*

SELECTED BIBLIOGRAPHY

Crislen C, Bahnson HT: Aneurysms of the aorta. Curr Probl Surg, December 1972

Mannick J (ed): Symposium on vascular surgery. Surg Clin North Am 59: 1979

Moore WS, Blaisdell FW: Diagnosis and management of peripheral arterial occlusive disease. Curr Probl Surg, November, 1973

Ross R, Glomset JA: The pathogenesis of atherosclerosis, two parts. New Engl J Med 295:369, 420, 1976

Stillman RM, Marino CA, Stillman BS: Vascular laboratory evaluation. In Sawyer PN, Stillman RM (eds): Vascular Diseases: Current Controversies. New York, Appleton-Century-Crofts, 1981, p 145

QUESTIONS

DIRECTIONS: The group of items below consists of five lettered headings, followed by a list of numbered phrases. For *each* numbered phrase, select the *one* lettered heading or lettered component that is most closely associated with it. Each lettered heading or lettered component may be selected once, more than once, or not at all.

A 65-year-old diabetic, hypertensive male with rest pain involving the toes of his right foot is found to have 95 percent stenosis of his right common iliac artery with essentially normal vasculature elsewhere. He is a smoker and has severe pulmonary emphysema.

        A   Aorto-(R) iliac bypass
        B   Aorto-(R) femoral bypass
        C   Femorofemoral crossover graft
        D   Aortobifemoral bypass
        E   (R) iliac endarterectomy

1. The safest reconstructive procedure for this patient?
2. Left iliac arterial flow least after which procedure?
3. Left iliac arterial flow greatest after which procedure?
4. Progression of disease in the left iliac artery is expected to be slowest after which procedure?
5. If distal atheroembolism is a problem and general anesthesia can be tolerated, what is the procedure of choice?

DIRECTIONS: Each of the questions or incomplete statements below is followed by five suggested answers or completions. Select the *one* that is *best* in each case.

---

6. A 50-year-old male with rest pain in his right foot and calf, and an arteriogram showing occlusion of his entire superficial femoral and popliteal vessels, with diffuse disease in the vessels of the leg will profit most by a(n):
   A. Reversed saphenous vein femoropopliteal bypass
   B. In-situ saphenous vein femoropopliteal bypass
   C. Composite graft
   D. Profundaplasty
   E. Bilateral lumbar sympathectomy
7. The most satisfactory graft material, in terms of patency rates, for femoropopliteal bypass grafting is:
   A. Autogenous saphenous vein
   B. Homologous saphenous vein
   C. Preserved bovine carotid artery
   D. Woven Dacron
   E. Knitted Dacron

A 69-year-old male with a pulsatile midabdominal mass is admitted for work-up.

8. The study *most likely* to correctly confirm the presence of an abdominal aortic aneurysm is:
   A. Sonography
   B. Abdominal lateral x-ray
   C. Physical examination
   D. Doppler
   E. Aortography

9. The patient is found to have a temperature of 100°F and a white cell count of 14,000/mm^3. If blood cultures grow Salmonella, the appropriate operative therapy after the administration of systemic antibiotics is:
   A. Aneurysmorraphy without synthetic graft
   B. Aneurysmectomy with aortic tube graft
   C. Aneurysmectomy with aortofemoral bypass graft
   D. Aneurysmectomy with axillofemoral bypass grafts
   E. Axillofemoral bypass with ligation of aneurysm

10. Assume that during laparotomy for a 6-cm asymptomatic abdominal aortic aneurysm, an almost obstructing carcinoma of the splenic flexure is discovered. The procedure of choice at that time is:
    A. Aneurysmectomy with bypass graft
    B. Aneurysmorraphy
    C. Left hemicolectomy
    D. Both aneurysmectomy and left hemicolectomy
    E. Aneurysmectomy and decompressive colostomy

11. A 75-year-old diabetic male with poor femoral pulses and no flow in the deep femoral artery develops sepsis and wet gangrene of the distal half of his left foot. No reconstruction was felt possible. The indicated immediate procedure is:
    A. Transmetatarsal amputation
    B. Standard B-K amputation
    C. Lumbar sympathectomy
    D. Physiologic or open amputation
    E. Standard A-K amputation

ANSWERS

1. **C** Can be performed under local anesthesia; percutaneous transluminal angioplasm should also be considered.
2. **D** Flow diverted through (L) limb of graft.
3. **C** Supplies both graft and donor site.
4. **C** Increased flow retards progression of atherosclerosis.
5. **E** Feasible only if discrete plaque and large diameter vessel without severe calcification.
6. **D** The profundaplasty is a quick procedure that may be performed under local anesthesia. Endarterectomy of the proximal vessels with patch graft will provide excellent collateral circulation around an occluded superficial femoral artery despite poor runoff. Absence of adequate

popliteal or leg vessel flow in this case will make femoropopliteal or femorotibial bypass impossible.

7. **A** To date, no graft material has been found to have patency rates comparable to autogenous saphenous vein in the femoropopliteal position.

8. **A** Sonography (echography) is virtually 100 percent accurate. Plainfilms of the abdomen are unreliable because only 50 percent are calcified. Physical exam is inaccurate because of the difficulty of differentiating tortuous aorta. Aortography visualizes only the lumen, which may be much smaller than the vessel that is occluded by thrombus.

9. **D** All infected tissue should be excised and extraanatomic bypass performed.

10. **C** Treat the lesion most likely to cause early problems first.

11. **D** Freezing (physiologic) or open (guillotine) amputation should be performed first. After patient is stabilized, he should have an A-K amputation because blood supply is inadequate to allow healing at the B-K level in this case.

20. Carotid

ANATOMY

1. Plaque is almost always segmental and at bifurcation
2. Intracranial vessels are usually free of disease

CLINICAL FINDINGS

1. Amaurosis fugax = transient monocular blindness
2. Retinal strokes (ophthalmic artery is branch of internal carotid)
3. Hemiparesis
4. Dysphasia
5. These may take the form of
   a. Transient ischemic attacks (TIA's), or
   b. Frank stroke

DIAGNOSIS

1. *Noninvasive*
   a. Listen for bruit at carotid bifurcation
   b. Phonoangiography
   c. Doppler (look for supraorbital artery flow reversal) (See Fig. 20-1)
   d. Brain scan (dynamic phase)
   e. Ultrasound imaging—requires high resolution
   f. Oculoplethysmography (plethysmodynamography)
   g. Digital subtraction angiography
2. *Invasive*
   a. Arteriography—aortic arch or by direct injection (See Fig. 20-2)

RESULTS OF PLAQUE AT BIFURCATION

1. Asymptomatic carotid bruit
2. Embolization of ulcerated plaque
3. Decrease in cerebral blood flow
4. Thrombosis and total occlusion of carotid

202

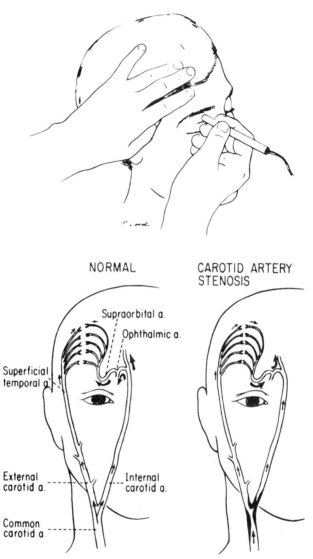

Figure 20-1 Reversal of flow in the supraorbital artery judged by a directional Doppler flow probe suggest stenosis of the ipsilateral internal carotid artery. *(From Haimovici H (ed): Vascular Surgery. Principles and Techniques. McGraw-Hill, 1976, pp 31 and 32, with permission.)*

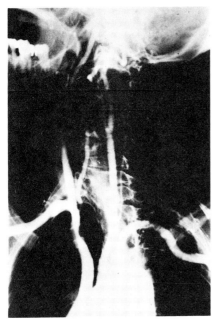 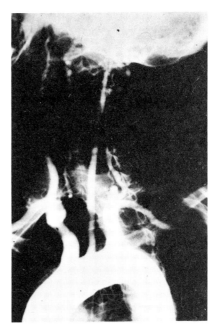

Figure 20-2   Carotid arteriogram showing normal vasculature (left), and one with total occlusion of the right internal carotid artery and narrowing of the left internal carotid artery (right).

INDICATIONS FOR CAROTID ENDARTERECTOMY

1. TIA
2. Preparation for major vascular surgery with existence of asymptomatic severe carotid stenosis
3. Chronic stroke
4. Acute stroke (delay at least three weeks)
5. Nonspecific neurologic signs
6. Asymptomatic bruit (debated)
7. Carotid aneurysm (rare)
8. Emergency endarterectomy for
   a. Stroke following angiography
   b. Postoperative stroke after endarterectomy

IF DISEASE IS BILATERAL

Symptomatic side first (independent of degree of narrowing), then wait and observe one month. If patient remains symptom-free, surgery *not* needed for contralateral side

TECHNIQUE

Prevention of Cerebral Ischemia During Clamping
1. Intraluminal shunt (Javid or other type)
2. Hypothermia
3. Hypertension
4. Hypercarbia
5. Diamox (carbonic anhydrase inhibitor)

Assessment of Adequacy of Back Flow
1. Preoperative arteriogram showing cross-filling of contralateral cerebral hemisphere
2. Neurologic evaluation with patient under local anesthesia
3. Carotid stump pressure measurements: if less than 50 mm Hg indicates need for shunt
4. Intraoperative EEG monitoring

Complications
1. Stroke (1 percent)
2. Death (usually due to associated diseases)
3. Severe hypertension in immediate postoperative period
4. False aneurysm (rare)
5. Bleeding

OTHER EXTRACRANIAL CEREBROVASCULAR DISEASE

1. *Vertebral artery occlusion:* If severely symptomatic, endarterectomy if possible (usually possible on right side), or end-to-side transposition of vertebral to carotid (usually required on left side)
2. *Carotid origin obstruction:* Thoracotomy avoided by end-to-side transposition to distal cervical portion of subclavian artery
3. *Subclavian steal syndrome* = proximal subclavian occlusion causing reversal of vertebral flow to supply ischemic upper extremity; treated with carotid-subclavian bypass

SELECTED BIBLIOGRAPHY

Thompson JE, Patman RD, Talkington CM: Carotid surgery for cerebrovascular insufficiency. Curr Probl Surg 15, 1978
Wylie EJ, Effeney DJ: Surgery of the aortic arch branches and vertebral diseases. Surg Clin North Am 59:669, 1979

QUESTIONS

DIRECTIONS: Each of the questions or incomplete statements below is followed by five suggested answers or completions. Select the *one* that is *best* in each case.

1. A 50-year-old male with episodes of transient blindness in his right eye requires aortofemoral bypass and left femoropopliteal bypass for severe claudication. Four-vessel angiography shows severe stenosis of both carotid bifurcations. The *first* operative procedure to be performed is:
   A. Aortofemoral bypass
   B. Left femoropopliteal bypass
   C. Right carotid endarterectomy
   D. Left carotid endarterectomy
   E. Bilateral carotid endarterectomy
2. During carotid endarterectomy, if a shunt is not used, assessment of adequacy of cerebral blood flow may be made by:
   A. EEG
   B. Measurement of carotid stump pressure
   C. Mental status under local anesthesia
   D. Preoperative arteriogram
   E. All of these
3. The patient most likely to benefit from carotid endarterectomy is one with:
   A. Transient cerebral ischemic attacks
   B. Total carotid occlusion
   C. An acute stroke
   D. A progressing stroke
   E. Vertibrobasilar symptoms
4. Transient ischemic attacks are usually due to:
   A. Total occlusion of the internal carotid artery
   B. Arterial emboli
   C. Total external carotid occlusion
   D. Transient hypotensive episodes with partial occlusion of the internal carotid artery
   E. None of these

DIRECTIONS: For each of the questions or incomplete statements below, *one* or *more* of the answers or completions given is correct. Select:

A   if only *1, 2, and 3* are correct
B   if only *1 and 3* are correct
C   if only *2 and 4* are correct
D   if only *4* is correct
E   if all are correct

---

5. Arch angiography is indicated in a patient with an asymptomatic bruit if:
   1. Aortofemoral bypass is to be performed
   2. There is reversal of supraorbital blood flow
   3. Bruits are bilateral and harsh
   4. Ophthalmodynamometry confirms decrease in flow
6. Emergency carotid endarterectomy is indicated for a(n):
   1. Cerebrovascular accident after arteriography

    2. Spontaneous acute stroke
    3. Cerebrovascular accident after carotid endarterectomy
    4. Retinal artery embolus
7. Methods used to increase cerebral blood flow intraoperatively:
    1. Hyperthermia
    2. Hypercarbia
    3. Hyperkalemia
    4. Hypertension
8. Structures which may require division during carotid endarterectomy:
    1. Hypoglossal nerve
    2. Superior thyroid artery
    3. Internal maxillary artery
    4. Common facial vein

ANSWERS

1. **C** Symptomatic side first. Doing bilateral endarterectomy at one sitting is fraught with danger.

2. **E** All of these.

3. **A** In series by DeWeese, 84 percent of patients improved after carotid endarterectomy if their symptomatology was classical TIA, while only 13 percent improved if their symptoms were nonclassical. Strokes will worsen unless at least three weeks are allowed before operation.

4. **B** Usually emboli from ulcerated plaque.

5. **E** Angiography may be indicated in all patients with bruits.

6. **B** Also, if bruit disappears in a hospitalized patient awaiting endarterectomy and in the presence of bilateral, severe carotid occlusion.

7. **C**

8. **C** Hypoglossal nerve and vagus nerve must be preserved.

21. Heart

CARDIOPULMONARY BYPASS

METHOD

1. Disposable bubble oxygenator (See Fig. 21-1)
2. Heparin: 300 units/kg; flow rates 50 ml/kg
3. Prime pump and tubing with acellular balanced salt solution → hemodilution → diminished red cell sludging
4. Hypothermia to ↓ metabolic demand

COMPLICATIONS

1. Cardiogenic shock due to:
   a. Coronary air emboli
   b. Damage to coronary artery
   c. Prolonged ischemia
   d. Underlying myocardial disease
   e. Hypovolemia due to third space loss
2. Postoperative hemorrhage—usually diffuse oozing due to inadequate reversal of heparin
3. Arrhythmia due to:
   a. Damage to conducting system
   b. Hypokalemia with digitalis toxicity
   c. Inadequate digitalis
4. Vascular damage
   a. While passing tape around aorta may damage major vessel (especially right branch of pulmonary artery). Control with digital pressure until dissection adequate for clamping
   b. Damage to coronary orifice. Avoided with hypothermia without coronary perfusion
   c. Intimal dissection in femoral cannulation
5. Peripheral embolization: air, or particulate matter (calcium, thrombi)
6. Hematologic damage
   a. Hemolysis—treat with mannitol diuresis
   b. Thrombocytopenia—platelets required
   c. Loss of clotting factors

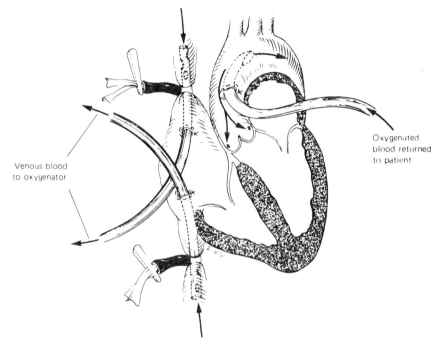

Venous blood
to oxygenator

Oxygenated
blood returned
to patient

Figure 21-1 Method of complete cardiopulmonary bypass. *(From Dunphy JE and Way LW (eds):* Current Surgical Diagnosis and Treatment. *3rd Edt. Lange, 1977, p 348, with permission).*

    d. Disseminated intravascular coagulopathy—due to inadequate heparinization

7. Renal insufficiency
8. Respiratory insuffuciency: due to platelet microemboli
9. Metabolic acidosis (lactic acidosis)
10. Postcardiotomy syndrome
    a. Clinical findings:
        i. Fever
        ii. Joint pains
        iii. Pericardial effusion
        iv. Pleural effusion
        v. Chest pain
        vi. Cardiac decompensation
    b. Interval: two weeks to three months postoperatively
    c. Etiology: unknown
    d. Therapy: salicylates, symptomatic, rarely steroids

CONGENITAL HEART DISEASE

ETIOLOGY

1. Idiopathic (usually)
2. Maternal rubella (1 to 2 percent)
   a. Patent ductus arteriosus
   b. Pulmonic stenosis
   c. Deafness
   d. Cataracts
3. Trisomy 21: persistent A-V canal

OCCURRENCE

Defect	Percent at birth
Ventricular septal defect	31
Atrial septal defect (ostium secundum mostly)	11
Pulmonic stenosis	9
Patent ductus arteriosus	8
Aortic stenosis	7
Coarctation of the aorta	6
Tetraology of Fallot	6
Transposition of the great vessels	5
Other	18

OVERALL CLASSIFICATION AND SEQUELAE

Defect	Sequelae	Examples	Treatment
Left-to-right shunt	(1) Pulmonary vascular congestion → Respiratory infections, insufficiency (2) Increased preload in involved ventricle → Concentric ventricular hypertrophy → Heart failure	(1) VSD (2) ASD (3) Patent ductus (4) Complete A-V canal (5) Total anomalous pulmonary venous connection	*Palliation—* Pulmonary artery banding *Definitive—* Closure of defect

(continued)

Defect	Sequelae	Examples	Treatment
Obstructive lesions	(1) 60% reduction in cross- sectional area → Systolic pressure difference across lesion → Turbulence & cavitation → Concentric hypertrophy of involved ventricle → Heart failure (2) Post-stenotic dilatation (3) Subacute bacterial endocarditis	(1) Pulmonic stenosis (2) Aortic stenosis (3) Coarctation of the aorta	Repair of lesion
Right-to- left shunt	(1) Obstructive lesion of (R) heart + septal defect → Redirection of pulmonary blood flow → Hypoxia, cyanosis → Polycythemia → Increased blood viscosity, dehydration, venous thrombosis, neurologic defects (2) (R) ventricular hypertrophy	(1) Tetralogy of Fallot	*Palliative*— Create systemic-pulmonary shunt *Definitive*— Correction of abnormality
Complex & rare malformation	Vary	(1) D-transposition of the great vessels	

ATRIAL SEPTAL DEFECT (OSTIUM PRIMUM) (L → R SHUNT)

Symptoms
1. Sometimes dyspnea on exertion, fatigue, heart failure

Signs
1. Systolic ejection murmur at (L) second intercostal space
2. Fixed split S_2
3. Systolic ejection murmur at apex radiating to axilla

EKG
1. (L) axis deviation
2. Prolonged P-R interval
3. Tall R-waves

Chest X-ray
1. Cardiomegaly
2. Increased pulmonary vasculature

Embryology
1. Incomplete formation of mitral and tricuspid valves and septa from endocardial cushions

Cardiac Catheterization
1. Increased O_2-saturation in RA
2. Increased LA pressure
3. Prominent v-wave
4. "Gooseneck" deformity of LV outflow tract

Complications
1. When associated with mitral or tricuspid regurgitation—CHF
2. Bacterial endocarditis
3. Pulmonary vascular disease in adulthood

Surgical Therapy
1. Repair with pericardial patch

Prognosis after Operation
1. Operative mortality 3 percent
2. Some patients develop complete heart block due to suture of conduction bundle

ATRIAL SEPTAL DEFECT (OSTIUM SECUNDUM) (L → R SHUNT)

Symptoms
1. Usually none
2. Rarely, heart failure

Signs
1. Midsystolic ejection murmur at upper (L) heart border
2. Fixed split S_2

EKG
1. Occasional (R) axis deviation and RVH

Chest X-ray
1. Increased pulmonary vascularity
2. Enlarged RA and RV

Lutembacher's Syndrome
1. Ostium secundum defect +   2. Mitral stenosis

Cardiac Catheterization
1. Catheter passes across atrial septum

Complications
1. Occur in adulthood   b. Pulmonic valvular disease
   a. Heart failure   c. Atrial arrhythmias

Indications for Surgery
1. L → R shunt greater than 2:1

Surgical Therapy
1. Closure by direct suture or patch

Prognosis after Operation
1. Operative mortality less than 1 percent

VENTRICULAR SEPTAL DEFECT (L → R SHUNT)

Symptoms
1. None if defect is small   4. Fatigue
2. Many close spontaneously   5. Feeding problems
3. Dyspnea on exertion

Signs
1. Pansystolic murmur with thrill along left sternal border
2. Hyperactive precordium
3. Soft, diastolic flow murmur at apex
4. Cardiomegaly
5. Hepatomegaly

EKG
1. Notched R-waves in V1-V3   2. LVH, RVH

Chest X-ray
1. Increased pulmonary vascularity   2. RVH, LVH

Cardiac Catheterization
1. Increased right ventricular O_2-saturation of over 10 percent
2. Catheter passes through defect

Complications
1. For large defects
   a. 5 percent die in infancy
   b. 25−40 percent defect decreases in size or closes
   c. 10 percent infundibular muscle hypertrophy with decreased pulmonary
      flow

d. 50 percent pulmonary vascular disease → flow across VSD balances or reverses (Eisenmenger's) → polycythemia, hypoxia, death by age 30−40

Medical Therapy
1. Many close spontaneously

Surgical Therapy
1. Close defect or patch
2. Close patent ductus in infants with CHF
3. Pulmonary artery banding in infants with complex defects

Prognosis after Operation
1. Right bundle branch block—50 percent
2. Permanent complete heart block—less than 1 percent
3. Operative mortality
   a. Banding 1−3 percent
   b. Total correction 15−30 percent if high pulmonary/systemic vascular resistance

PATENT DUCTUS ARTERIOSUS (L → R SHUNT)

Symptoms
1. Usually none
2. Feeding problems
3. Heart failure
4. Enterocolitis
5. Dyspnea

Signs
1. Hepatomegaly
2. Continuous (machinery) murmur in (L) second intercostal space
3. Increased LV impulse
4. Loud S_2
5. Widened pulse pressure
6. Bounding peripheral pulses

EKG
1. Usually normal

Chest X-ray
1. Increased pulmonary vascularity
2. Prominent PA
3. LVH

Embryology
1. Normally closes by three months of age by constriction of smooth muscle which starts within first few days of life

Cardiac Catheterization
1. Catheter passes through ductus
2. Increased pulmonary artery pressure
3. Increased O_2 saturation in PA
4. Echocardiogram may establish diagnosis

Complications
1. Associated with respiratory distress syndrome in premature infants
2. Subacute bacterial endocarditis
3. Cardiac failure

Medical Therapy
1. Prostaglandin E_1 inhibitor (Indomethacin) may cause closure of patent ductus in infants

Surgical therapy
1. Ligation by extrathoracic route
2. Indicated if medical therapy fails
3. Contraindicated if shunt is balanced or reversed (i.e., R → L)

Prognosis after Operation
1. Operative mortality 0.2 percent in uncomplicated cases

COMPLETE ATRIOVENTRICULAR CANAL (L → R SHUNT)

Symptoms
1. Heart failure early in life
2. Poor feeding
3. Failure to thrive
4. Respiratory problems

Signs
1. Tachypnea
2. Hepatomegaly
3. Blowing pansystolic murmur and thrill at left sternal border
4. Fixed split S_2

EKG
1. Left axis deviation
2. RVH, LVH
3. Prolonged P-R interval

Chest X-ray
1. Cardiomegaly
2. Increased pulmonary vascularity
3. Pulmonary congestion

Definition
1. Direct communication between two ventricles; mitral and tricuspid valves fused

Cardiac Catheterization
1. Arterialized blood in RA
2. Catheter easily passes into all chambers
3. Increased pulmonary vascular resistance
4. "Gooseneck" deformity of mitral valve and LV outflow tract

Complications
1. Heart failure
2. Respiratory infections
3. Death

Surgical Therapy
1. Banding of pulmonary artery for pulmonary hypertension
2. Complete repair if pulmonary vascular resistance is less than 70 percent of systemic vascular resistance

Prognosis after Operation
1. Complete heart block 5–10 percent   3. Late deaths 5–10 percent
2. Operative mortality
   a. 20 percent in infants
   b. 5–15 percent thereafter

TOTAL ANOMALOUS PULMONARY VENOUS CONNECTION (L → R SHUNT)

Symptoms
1. Minimal cyanosis
2. Heart failure
3. Poor feeding
4. Dyspnea
5. Fatigue
6. Failure to thrive

Signs
1. Prominent RV heave
2. Hepatomegaly
3. Loud S_2
4. Pulmonic flow murmur
5. Gallop rhythm

EKG
1. (R) axis deviation
2. (R) atrial hypertrophy
3. RVH

Chest X-ray
1. "Snowman" (figure-of-eight) pattern due to two superior vena cavas

Classification
1. Pulmonary veins → common vein → RA (55 percent)
2. Pulmonary veins → coronary sinus → RA (30 percent)
3. Pulmonary veins → common pulmonary vein →
4. Inferior vena cava, portal vein or ductus venosus (12 percent)

Surgical Therapy
1. Balloon atrial septostomy via cardiac catheterization if associated ASD is insufficient
2. Emergency correction if seriously ill

Prognosis after Operation
1. Operative mortality
   a. 30−50 percent under 3 months
   b. 5 percent in older children

PULMONIC STENOSIS (OBSTRUCTIVE LESION)

Symptoms
1. Mild: none
2. Severe: cyanosis, dyspnea, hypoxia, angina, syncope
3. Angina
4. Syncope
5. Feeding problems

Signs
1. High-pitched systolic ejection murmur at left second intercostal space
2. S_2 delayed, soft
3. Ejection click

EKG
1. RAH, RVH

Chest X-ray
1. Dilated PA
2. RVH

Classification
1. Valvular 95 percent
2. Infundibular 5 percent

Cardiac Catheterization
1. Increased pulmonary vascular resistance

Indications for Surgery
1. Infants with RV failure, hypoxia, or if pressure difference greater than 60 mm Hg across valve

Surgical Therapy
1. Open valvulotomy with closure of foramen ovale, patent ductus or ASD if present

Prognosis after Operation
1. Operative mortality 2−3 percent
2. Residual abnormalities 10 percent

AORTIC VALVULAR STENOSIS (OBSTRUCTIVE LESION)

Symptoms
1. Usually none
2. Dyspnea

Signs
1. Harsh systolic murmur at base
2. Prominent LV impulse
3. Narrow pulse pressure
4. Hepatomegaly

EKG
1. LVH
2. Correlates better with vectorcardiogram

Chest X-ray
1. Pulmonary venous congestion
2. Poststenotic dilatation of ascending aorta

Classification
1. Valvular (most common)
2. Subaortic
3. Supravalvular
4. Asymmetric septal hypertrophy

Cardiac Catheterization
1. To differentiate from other causes of AS and to delineate associated anomalies

Complications
1. Sudden death 1–7 percent
2. Bacterial endocarditis

Medical Therapy
1. Digitalis, diuretics

Surgical Therapy
1. Commissurotomy if not responsive to medical therapy or if systolic pressure gradient greater than 50 mm Hg

Prognosis after Operation
1. Elective operative mortality 5 percent
2. Late deaths 10 percent
3. Reoperation required 25 percent

COARCTATION OF THE AORTA (OBSTRUCTIVE LESION)

Symptoms
1. Usually none
2. Headaches
3. Fatigue
4. Epistaxis
5. Claudication

Signs
1. Weak femoral pulses
2. Elevated brachial pressure
3. Harsh systolic murmur at left sternal border

EKG
1. LVH

Chest X-ray
1. LV enlargement
2. Notched ribs T3-T8 (collaterals)
3. "3" sign on chest x-ray or "E" sign on esophagogram = bulging aorta proximal and distal to coarctation

Classification
1. Diaphragmlike constriction just distal to left subclavian with poststenotic dilatation; if associated with patent ductus arteriosus = preductal or infantile type, mortality is high

Cardiac Catheterization
1. Documents length of segment and associated anomalies such as aberrant (R) subclavian artery

Complications
1. Death in infancy or before age 40 from heart failure, cerebral hemorrhage or thrombosis, dissecting aneurysm

Medical Therapy
1. Digoxin, diuretics,
2. Morphine, oxygen
3. (Allow postponement of operation until childhood)

Surgical Therapy
1. Resection with or without interposition graft; best if performed between 4 and 8 years of age

Prognosis after Operation
1. Elective: Operative mortality 1–2 percent
2. Emergency: Operative mortality 15–25 percent
3. Complications
   a. Hemorrhage
   b. Paraplegia (rare)
   c. Abdominal pain (common)
   d. Paradoxical hypertension due to sympathetic overactivity
   e. Recurrent coarctation is a problem in infants

TETRALOGY OF FALLOT (R → L SHUNT)

Symptoms
1. Cyanosis
2. Feeding problems
3. Fatigue
4. Hyperventilation
5. Hypoxic spells
6. Squatting
7. Neurologic defects

Signs
1. Systolic murmur at left sternal border

EKG
1. RVH

Chest X-ray
1. "Sabot"-shaped heart
2. Decreased pulmonary vascularity
3. RVH
4. (R) sided arch (20 percent)

Definition
1. Hypoplastic infundibulum with pulmonary artery obstruction
2. Overriding aorta
3. Large ventricular septal defect
4. Right ventricular hypertrophy

Cardiac Catheterization
1. Right-to-left shunt

Complications
1. Death in infancy or by age 20 from hypoxia, infection, or complications of polycythemia

Surgical Therapy (debated)
1. Total correction, or
2. Palliative shunt
3. Blalock-Taussig (subclavian to pulmonary artery)-*preferred*
4. Waterston (aortic to right pulmonary artery)-*flow difficult to control*
5. Potts (descending aorta to left pulmonary artery)-*difficult to close*

Prognosis after Operation
1. Operative mortality
   a. Shunt: less than 5 percent
   b. Correction: 5 percent
   c. If previous shunt: 10 percent

TRANSPOSITION OF THE GREAT VESSELS (COMPLEX MALFORMATION)

Symptoms and Signs
1. Intact ventricular septum → cyanosis at birth, which increases when ductus closes
2. VSD → less severe symptoms
3. Later → polycythemia, hepatomegaly, cardiomegaly

EKG
1. Normal or RVH, LVH

Chest X-ray
1. Egg-shaped heart
2. (R) sided aorta
3. Cardiomegaly
4. Congested lungs

Definition
1. Aorta arising from RV,
2. Pulmonary artery from LV
3. Survival depends on associated PDA or septal defect

Cardiac Catheterization
1. Systemic pressure in RV
2. Catheter passes directly into aorta from RV

Complications
1. 50 percent of infants die by 1 month
2. 90 percent die within 1 year

Medical Therapy
1. Digoxin, oxygen

Surgical Therapy
1. Balloon catheter atrial septostomy (Rashkind procedure) in infants
2. Mustard operation—baffle inserted in atrium to redirect venous blood through mitral valve
3. Right ventricular patch
4. Anatomic correction with transfer of ostia of coronary arteries

Prognosis after Operation
1. Mustard procedure mortality
   a. 5−10 percent if no VSD
   b. 20−30 percent is associated VSD
2. Supraventricular arrhythmias common

ACQUIRED HEART DISEASE

VALVULAR DISEASES

MITRAL STENOSIS

Symptoms
1. Failure
2. Hemoptysis
3. Chest pain

Signs
1. Accentuated mitral first sound
2. Loud opening snap
3. Increased P_2
4. Low-pitched diastolic murmur with presystolic accentuation

EKG
1. Atrial fibrillation
2. Increased P wave due to LA hypertrophy

Chext X-ray
1. Prominent LA appendage & PA
2. Calcific deposits on valve
3. Kerley "B" lines = lymphatic engorgement in lung periphery

Etiology
1. Usually rheumatic fever   2. Congenital is rare

Cardiac Catheterization
1. Increased PA and wedge pressures rising with exercise

Complications
1. Atrial fibrillation
2. Atrial thromboemboli
3. Cardiac asthma

Medical Therapy
1. Digitalis   3. Diuretics
2. Quinidine   4. Salt restriction

Indications for Commissurotomy
1. Any symptoms

Indications for Valve Replacement
1. Recurrent stenosis after commissurotomy
2. Patients over 55
3. Heavily calcified valve
4. Association with aortic disease requiring valve replacement

Prognosis
1. Recurrence usual after commissurotomy
2. Atrial fibrillation reversible in less than one-third of patients
3. Operative mortality: 1 to 8 percent

MITRAL INSUFFICIENCY

Symptoms
1. Insidious
2. Occur late
3. Fatigue, CHF

Signs
1. LV heave
2. Apical systolic murmur

EKG
1. Atrial fibrillation

Chest X-ray
1. Prominent LA
2. LVH
3. Kerley "B" lines

Etiology
1. Rheumatic fever
2. Myxomatous degeneration
3. Attenuation of subvalvular structures
4. Rupture of chordae tendineae or papillary muscles
5. Myocardiopathy
6. Bacterial endocarditis

Catheterization
1. Increased LA pressure
2. High V wave
3. Regurgitation of contrast on cineangiography

Complications
1. Atrial fibrillation
2. Congestive heart failure

Medical Therapy
1. Digitalis
2. Diuretics
3. Salt restriction

Indications for Valve Replacement
1. Progressive disability   2. Cardiomegaly

Prognosis
1. LV function may be impaired for months postoperatively
2. Operative mortality: 5 to 10 percent

AORTIC STENOSIS

Symptoms
1. *Minimal until terminal phase*
   a. Syncope
   b. Angina on exertion
   c. Failure

Signs
1. Diamond-shaped systolic ejection murmur in the (R) second interspace radiating to neck
2. Diminished peripheral pulses
3. Peripheral vasoconstriction

EKG
1. LVH
2. Atrial fibrillation in late stages

Chest X-ray
1. LVH in long-standing disease
2. Sometimes calcified valve

Etiology
1. Rheumatic fever (30 to 50 percent)
2. Superimposed calcification on congenital stenosis

Cardiac Catheterization
1. LV systolic pressure > aortic systolic pressure
2. Increased LV end-diastolic pressure in advanced cases
3. Anacrotic notch on aortic pressure curve
4. Difficult passage thru aortic valve may require transseptal or percutaneous route

Complications
1. Sudden death due to V-fibrillation

Medical Therapy
1. None

Indications for Valve Replacement
1. Any symptoms

Prognosis
1. Operative mortality: 5 percent   2. Late mortality: 1 to 3 percent yearly

AORTIC INSUFFICIENCY

Symptoms
1. Failure that may occur late especially if disease develops slowly

Signs
1. Diminished arterial diastolic pressure, increasing as disease worsens
2. Blowing diastolic murmur at LSB

EKG
1. LVH

Chest X-ray
1. LVH   2. Pulmonary congestion

Etiology
1. Rheumatic fever (70 to 80 percent)   5. Marfan's syndrome
2. Bacterial endocarditis   6. Rheumatoid arthritis
3. Syphilis   7. Congenital (rare)
4. Dissecting aneurysm

Cardiac Catheterization
1. Increased wedge pressure
2. Delayed dicrotic notch

Complications
1. Impaired coronary flow due to decreased diastolic pressure
2. Embolization from bacterial vegetation

Medical Therapy
1. Digitalis

Indications for Valve Replacement
1. LV end-diastolic pressure over 15 mm Hg with first evidence of failure

Prognosis
1. Operative mortality: < 5 percent

TRICUSPID DISEASE

Symptoms
1. Usually minimal, as even complete tricuspid excision is well tolerated

Signs
1. Hepatomegaly
2. Edema
3. Ascites
4. Elevated venous pressure
5. Pulsatile liver

Chest X-ray
1. RA hypertrophy

Etiology
1. Usually associated with mitral or aortic disease

Cardiac Catheterization
1. Increased RA pressure with high V wave
2. Exceptions:
    a. Bacterial endocarditis with narcotic addiction or tumor (example carcinoid)

Complications
1. Endocarditis

Medical Therapy
1. Digitalis
2. Diuretics
3. Salt restriction

Indications for Valve Replacement
1. Usually only advanced disease and during replacement of other valves
2. Annuloplasty may be possible
3. Complete excision for bacterial endocarditis

Prognosis
1. Operative mortality: 10 to 15 percent (due to multivalvular disease)

CORONARY ARTERY DISEASE

Clinical Findings
1. Substernal chest pain on exertion, exposure to cold or emotion. May radiate to arm, neck, or jaw. Relieved by rest or nitroglycerine
2. Variant (Prinzmetal's angina) = chest pain at rest, not exercise. ST elevation found during attacks
3. Congestive heart failure

4. Associated factors
   a. Hypertension
   b. Hypercholesterolemia
   c. Family history of coronary artery disease
   d. Earlobe creases

Diagnosis
1. EKG—ST depression on exercising, evidence of previous myocardial infarction
2. Perfusion imaging—scan with Thallium 201
3. Lactate metabolism—abnormal during atrial pacing
4. Angiography—with LV cineangiography to determine LV function

Medical Therapy
1. Nitroglycerine (short-acting)
2. Isosorbide dinitrate (long-acting)
3. Propranolol (beta-blocker)
4. Stop smoking
5. Treat underlying problems
   a. Hyperlipidemia
   b. Hypertension
   c. Overweight

Surgical Therapy
1. Indications for coronary bypass
   a. Disabling symptoms unresponsive to medical therapy
   b. Unstable or preinfarction angina
   c. Postmyocardial infarction angina
   d. Myocardial ischemia without angina
   e. Myocardial infarction in patient under 45 years old
   f. At valve replacement
2. Requirements for reconstructability
   a. Greater than 70 percent stenosis of at least one major coronary artery
   b. Satisfactory distal vessels
   c. Acceptable left ventricular function
   d. *Not* within six weeks of acute myocardial infarction
3. Procedure
   a. Aortocoronary bypass (on cardiopulmonary bypass)
      i. Saphenous vein (usual)
      ii. Prosthetic graft
   b. Internal mammary anastomosis to coronary artery
   c. Coronary endarterectomy with patch graft
4. Complications
   a. Atherosclerosis in graft
   b. Mortality 4 percent up to 30 days postoperatively—depends on LV function

   c. No relief in 10 to 40 percent
   d. Graft occlusion—15 to 30 percent at one year
5. Indications for emergency coronary bypass
   a. Acute myocardial infarction while awaiting bypass or during catheterization
   b. Acute MI or cardiogenic shock (debated)

Factors Associated with Poor Prognosis

1. Sex (early mortality twice as high in females)
2. Advanced age
3. Poor left ventricular function
4. Diffuse coronary disease
5. Advanced functional status
6. Serious associated disease
7. High left ventricular end-diastolic pressure
8. Prior congestive heart failure
9. Myocardial infarction within one week prior to operation
10. Stenosis of left main coronary vessel

CARDIAC TRANSPLANTATION

1. Indication: ischemic heart disease or cardiopyopathy; when no other therapy is possible
2. Technique: atrium transected so that entries of vena cavae and pulmonary veins remain *in situ*
3. Immunosuppression: steroids, antilymphocyte globulin, Cyclosporin A
4. Prognosis:
   a. 50 percent 5-year survival
   b. High pulmonary vascular resistance decreases survival rate
5. Heterotopic cardiac transplant
   a. Advantage: both hearts can work simultaneously; especially good if pulmonary vascular resistance is high
   b. Disadvantage: difficult to diagnose early rejection
6. Implanted artificial heart
   a. Indication: terminal cardiac failure and transplantation impossible
   b. Prognosis: unknown; first human implant (Jarvik-7) by DeVries in late 1982

DISSECTING AORTIC ANEURYSMS

	Ascending	Descending
Age group	Younger	Older
Associated findings	Marfan's syndrome	Hypertension
	Cystic medial necrosis	Generalized atherosclerosis

(continued)

	Ascending	Descending
Clinical findings	Anterior chest pain Pulse deficit Aortic insufficiency Congestive heart failure Neurologic deficits	Interscapular back pain
Treatment	Immediate surgery: death from rupture of false lumen into pericardium or acute aortic insufficiency	Propranolol (decreases shearing force of left ventricular stroke volume). Intravenous nitroprusside or trimethaphan (decreases pulse pressure to 40 mmHg and mean BP to 90 mmHg, but maintains organ perfusion)
Mortality	25 percent with surgery	25 percent without surgery, one-third of patients will require elective operation because of increase in size

SELECTED BIBLIOGRAPHY

Behrendt DM, Austen WG: Patient Care in Cardiac Surgery, 2nd Edt. New York, Little Brown, 1976

Kirklin JW, Pacifico AD: Surgery for acquired valvular heart disease, two parts. N Engl J Med 288:133, 194, 1973

Pudolph AM: Congenital Heart Disease. Chicago, Yearbook Medical Publishers, 1974

QUESTIONS

1. One month after mitral valve replacement, a 27-year-old female returns with chest and joint pain, fever, and right pleural effusion. Blood cultures are negative. The most likely problem is:
   A. Failure of valve
   B. Involvement of aortic valve
   C. Peripheral embolization
   D. Postcardiotomy syndrome
   E. Sepsis

2. The common great vessel to sustain inadvertent injury during open heart surgery is the:
   A. Aorta
   B. Superior vena cava
   C. Inferior vena cava
   D. Pulmonary artery
   E. Pulmonary vein

A premature infant with respiratory distress syndrome and feeding problems is noted by his pediatrician to have a continuous murmur loudest in the second left intercostal space. Chest x-ray reveals increased pulmonary vascularity, left ventricular enlargement, and prominent pulmonary arteries.

3. The most likely defect is:
   A. Tetralogy of Fallot
   B. Transposition of the great vessels
   C. Aortic stenosis
   D. Ventricular septal defect
   E. Patent ductus arteriosus
4. Initial therapy for this defect is:
   A. Valve replacement
   B. Mustard procedure
   C. Ligation
   D. Pulmonary artery banding
   E. Medical

A six-year-old female is found on routine physical examination to have a systolic murmur throughout the precordium. Chest x-ray reveals moderate left ventricular hypertrophy. Blood pressures are recorded as follows:

Right arm	90/50
Left arm	165/95
Right leg	85/60
Left leg	85/60

5. The most likely diagnosis is:
   A. Patent ductus arteriosus
   B. Tetralogy of Fallot
   C. Preductal coarctation of the aorta
   D. Postductal coarctation of the aorta
   E. Coarctation of the aorta associated with anomalous right subclavian artery
6. After excision and correction of the anomaly, the blood pressure should be expected to:
   A. Rise temporarily, then fall to normal levels
   B. Fall immediately and remain at normal levels
   C. Fall slowly over several weeks to normal levels
   D. Remain elevated until adulthood
   E. Show no change
7. If the blood pressure rises postoperatively and the patient complains of abdominal pain, appropriate therapy should include:
   A. Reoperation and revision of graft
   B. Cardiac catheterization
   C. Exploratory laparotomy
   D. Sympathetic blocking agents
   E. No specific therapy
8. Absence of cyanosis in a newborn with the Tetralogy of Fallot may be due to:
   A. Polycythemia
   B. Anemia
   C. Patent ductus arteriosus

D. Hyperventilation

E. Right ventricular hypertrophy

9. Patent ductus arteriosus is most often diagnosed by:
    A. Chest x-ray
    B. Failure to thrive
    C. Machinery murmur
    D. EKG
    E. Dyspnea on exertion

10. Ligation of a patent ductus arteriosus is contraindicated in the presence of:
    A. Left-to-right shunt
    B. Cardiomegaly
    C. Right-to-left shunt
    D. Polycythemia
    E. None of these

11. Nonoperative therapy of patent ductus arteriosus is by inhibition of:
    A. Growth hormone
    B. Thyroid function
    C. Beta-H receptors
    D. Prostaglandin E_1
    E. Pituitary function

12. Asymptomatic patients with patent ductus arteriosus should have ligation:
    A. When first diagnosed
    B. In infancy
    C. By age 4 to 5 years
    D. As adults
    E. Never

13. Indications for surgical intervention in the Tetralogy of Fallot:
    A. When diagnosed
    B. Cyanosis at rest
    C. Cyanosis during exercise
    D. Anoxemia
    E. In adulthood

14. Indications for surgical intervention in infantile coarctation of the aorta:
    A. When diagnosed
    B. At age 4 to 5 years
    C. After puberty
    D. When pulmonary hypertension occurs
    E. When subacute bacterial endocarditis occurs

15. The usual treatment of ventricular septal defect in infants:
    A. Balloon atrial septostomy
    B. Blalock-Taussig shunt
    C. Pulmonary artery banding
    D. Anatomic correction
    E. Medical

16. The most common cause of cyanotic congenital heart disease is:
    A. Ventricular septal defect
    B. Ostium secundum defect

C. Transposition of the great vessels
D. Tetralogy of Fallot
E. Patent ductus arteriosus

17. The most serious threat to life in adults with congenital heart disease is:
    A. Myocardial infarction
    B. Pulmonary embolism
    C. Subacute bacterial endocarditis
    D. Malignant hypertension
    E. Congestive heart failure

18. The most common etiology of arrhythmia following open heart surgery is:
    A. Atrial trauma
    B. Myocardial infarction
    C. Air embolism to coronaries
    D. Electrolyte imbalance
    E. Hypotension

19. The most commonly used procedure in the operative treatment of coronary artery occlusive disease is:
    A. Coronary endarterectomy
    B. Implantation of internal mammary artery into myocardium
    C. Bovine aortocoronary bypass
    D. Dacron aortocoronary bypass
    E. Autogenous saphenous vein aortocoronary bypass

20. The highest *overall* operative mortality is in:
    A. Mitral valve replacement
    B. Aortic valve replacement
    C. Closed mitral commissurotomy
    D. Tricuspid valve replacement
    E. Open mitral commisurotomy

ANSWERS

1. **D** Postcardiotomy syndrome occurs two weeks to three months after cardiopulmonary bypass, is of unknown etiology, and is treated with salicylates or steroids.

2. **D** Injury to the right branch of the pulmonary artery may occur while passing the tape around the aorta.

3. **E**

4. **E** A continuous (machinery) murmur in the left second interspace suggests patent ductus arteriosus. This is often associated with respiratory distress syndrome in premature infants. Indomethacin (an inhibitor of prostaglandin E_1) may provoke closure of the patent ductus in infants. If it fails, ligation will be necessary.

5. **E**

6. **C**

7. **D** Weak femoral pulses with elevated brachial pressures suggests coarctation of the aorta. Cardiac catheterization is necessary to rule out

associated anomalies, as in this case where the diminished blood pressure in the right arm is due to an anomalous right subclavian artery which arises beyond the obstruction. If possible, operation should be postponed until childhood (age 4 to 8) because of the incidence of recurrent coarctation in infants requiring operation. Postoperatively, the blood pressure usually shows a slow decline over a period of weeks, but paradoxical hypertension and abdominal pain may occur and are due to sympathetic overactivity. Treatment is with sympathetic blocking agents.

8. **C** Absence of cyanosis in a newborn with the Tetralogy of Fallot may be due to a patent ductus arteriosus, which will help to overcome the right-to-left shunt.

9. **C** A machinery murmur is characteristic of a patent ductus arteriosus.

10. **C** When severe pulmonary damage results from a patent ductus arteriosus, pulmonary hypertension may eventually cause a reversal of flow in the shunt. In this case, ligation of the patent ductus would worsen the disease.

11. **D** Indomethacin is an inhibitor of prostaglandin E_1 and may cause closure of a patent ductus in infancy.

12. **C** Asymptomatic patients with patent ductus arteriosus should have it closed by age 4 to 5 years. Risks if it is left open include SBE and cardiac failure, so that life expectancy is 20 to 30 years if not ligated.

13. **D** Patients tend to tolerate the Tetralogy of Fallot rather well and operation may be postponed to allow definitive rather than palliative correction. However, the onset of anoxemia, especially when associated with growth retardation, is an indication for operative intervention.

14. **D** Coarctation of the aorta is best corrected between ages 4 and 8 years because of the high incidence of recurrent coarctation if the operation is performed in infancy. Medical therapy may allow postponement of surgery, but pulmonary hypertension is an indication for operative repair.

15. **E** Ventricular septal defects often regress and close spontaneously.

16. **D** The most common form of congenital heart disease is ventricular septal defect; however the commonest form of *cyanotic* congenital heart disease is the Tetralogy of Fallot.

17. **C** In adults with congenital heart disease, 40 percent of deaths result from subacute bacterial endocarditis. The next most frequent cause is cardiac failure.

18. **A** It is known that in open heart cases where the atrium is entered, the incidence of arrhythmia is significantly greater.

19. **E** Aortocoronary bypass using the saphenous vein is the procedure of choice today. Preserved arteries, veins and prosthetic materials are inferior.

20. **D** The high operative mortality in tricuspid valve procedures results from commonly associated disease in aortic and/or mitral valves.

22. Veins and Thromboembolism

VEINS

ANATOMY

Superficial Veins
1. Greater saphenous: anterior to medial malleolus → fossa ovalis → femoral vein
2. Lesser saphenous: posterior to lateral malleolus → popliteal vein

Perforators
1. Three posterosuperior to medial malleolus
2. Carry blood from deep to superficial system
3. Normally valves prevent reverse flow

Flow in Veins Results from
1. *Vis à tergo* (force from behind)
2. Muscular action
3. Respiration (?)
4. Forward flow guaranteed by valves

PATHOGENESIS OF VENOUS THROMBOSIS (See Fig. 22-1)

1. In general (Virchow's triad)
   a. Stasis
   b. Intimal damage
   c. Hypercoagulability
2. Specifically
   a. Stasis (bed rest, sitting, prolonged standing, illness, trauma, immobilization) → accumulation of thrombin → initiation of platelet .aggregation and release of platelet factor III → further increase in thrombin production → fibrin formation
   b. Intimal damage → release of thromboplastins → activation of *extrinsic* clotting system
   c. Intimal damage → activation of factor XII → triggering of *intrinsic* clotting system (See Fig. 22-2)

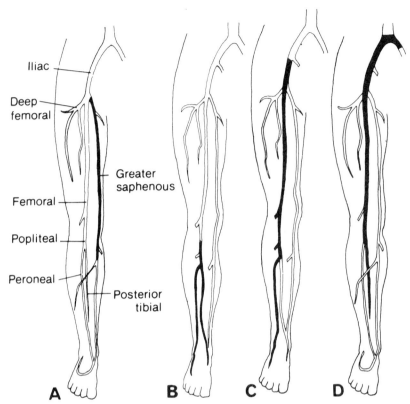

Figure 22-1 Common patterns of venous thrombosis. Superficial thrombophlebitis (A), most common form of deep venous thrombosis (B), extensive deep venous thrombosis, which may cause phlegmasia alba dolens or phlegmasia cerulea dolens (C, D).

    d. Intimal trauma and stasis → local hypercoagulability → thrombosis extending to normal vessels

    e. Evidence that "L" forms (especially of *Bacteroides*) growing from thrombi produce *Heparinase* (suggest tetracycline in therapy)

CLINICAL COURSE

1. Venous thrombosis: pain, swelling, redness, tenderness, tachycardia
2. Distal venous hypertension: edema, venous gangrene (if venous pressure greater than local arterial pressure)
3. Recanalization may occur: but leads to destruction of valves, varicose veins
4. Secondary varicose veins; edema, brawny induration, brownish discoloration (hemosiderin), dermatitis, ulceration (usually posterosuperior to malleoli)
5. Night cramps due to sustained contraction of muscles (etiology unknown)
6. Loose thrombi → pulmonary emboli (unlikely if thrombus confined to calf)

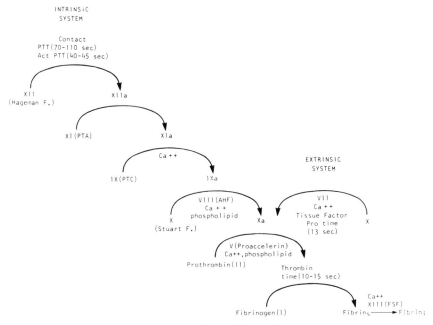

Figure 22-2   Coagulation pathways.

DIAGNOSIS

1. Clinical signs—notoriously unreliable
2. Venography (See Fig. 22-3) — *the* definitive test
   a. Constant filling defect
   b. Abrupt termination of column of contrast at constant site
   c. Nonfilling of deep system
   d. Diversion of flow (collaterals to deep system)
   e. Varicose veins, incompetent perforators
3. I-125 fibrinogen scanning
   a. Incorporates into thrombus
   b. Expectant use: inject preop, scan periodically postop
   c. Diagnostic use: reliable only in propagating thrombus
   d. Overall, 90 percent correlation with phlebography
   e. Problems:
      i. Transmission of serum hepatitis
      ii. Unreliable in upper thigh and pelvis due to background counts in pelvic area
      iii. False positives in hematoma, cellulitis, arthritis, edema, wounds
4. Doppler ultrasound
   a. Absence of venous flow signals
   b. Loss of respiratory fluctuations

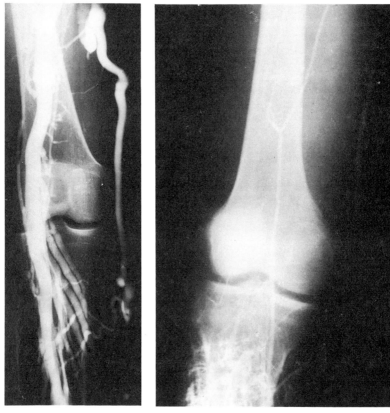

Figure 22-3 Normal ascending venogram (left), and one showing a constant filling defect and collateralization around the thrombosed deep venous system (right).

     c. Diminished augmentation of flow velocity resulting from compression of distal limb

     d. Lack of bilateral symmetry

     e. Good screening procedure, but high incidence of false positives and negatives

5. Plethysmography and Doppler ultrasound: 70 to 90 percent accuracy; subjective

     a. Difficult to perform

6. Rule out occult malignancy in thrombophlebitis migrans

SPECIAL PROBLEMS IN PREGNANT PATIENT

1. Edema and pain, even unilateral, may occur in absence of thrombosis

2. Must avoid fetal exposure to x-rays; hence, only limited venogram possible

3. Anticoagulation may be hazardous; coumadin contradicted because it passes placenta
4. I-131 fibrinogen scan contradicted
5. Plethysmography and Doppler studies may be inaccurate because of extrinsic compression of intraabdominal veins

THERAPY

Deep Venous Thrombosis
1. Heparin to keep partial thromboplastin time (PTT) 2 to 2.5 times normal
   a. Intermittent or continuous intravenous heparin for inpatients
   b. Subcutaneous heparin (20 to 40,000 units s/c daily) for outpatients (controversial)—allows ambulation, thereby preventing further stasis
   c. Coumadin (orally): high incidence of bleeding except low dose coumadin—promising new concept
2. Elevation of legs while in bed
3. Elastic stockings or wraps
4. Avoid prolonged sitting or standing
5. Avoid dehydration
6. Venous thrombectomy: only for ileofemoral thrombosis with phlegmasia cerulea dolens → arterial inflow compromised

Varicose Veins
1. *Nonoperative:* elevation while in bed, exercise, external support
2. *Operative:* indicated only if NO evidence of deep venous thrombosis; for chronic venous stasis ulcer, intractability, cosmesis, bleeding, recurrent superficial phlebitis
   a. *Ligation:* must ligate exactly at saphenofemoral junction, and transect all four branches in groin (lateral femoral cutaneous vein often missed)
   b. *Linton procedure* = subfascial ligation of incompetent perforating veins
   c. *Injection sclerotherapy:* for minor or recurrent varicosities

Chronic Venous Hypertension (postphlebitic syndrome)
1. *Nonoperative:* elevation while in bed, exercise, external support, local care of ulcers
2. *Operative:* indicated for intractable edema or ulceration
   a. Crossover saphenous bypass (Palma procedure): for unilateral iliac vein occlusion
   b. Valvular repair or valve transposition: new procedure, long-term results unknown

Superficial Phlebitis
1. Rule out associated deep venous thrombosis
2. Treat wiith warm compresses, antibiotics (?)
3. If suppurative, involved vein must be EXCISED

PULMONARY EMBOLISM

INCIDENCE IN HOSPITALIZED PATIENTS

1. Fatal—1/200
2. Nonfatal—1/100
3. Asymptomatic—as high as 10 to 20 percent

DIAGNOSIS

Symptoms and Signs (A sizable number have no definite signs)
(In decreasing order of frequency)
1. Tachypnea
2. Dyspnea
3. Pleuritic chest pain
4. Apprehension
5. Cough
6. Hemoptysis
7. Shock
8. Pleural friction rub
9. Clinical evidence of deep venous thrombosis

Bloods
(In decreasing order of frequency)
1. Decreased Po_2
2. Increased DHL
3. Leukocytosis
4. Increased SGOT
5. Increased bilirubin

EKG (uncommon)
1. Acute right-axis shift
2. S1/Q3/T3 pattern
3. Incomplete RBBB

Chest X-ray
1. Pulmonary infiltrate
2. Pleural effusion
3. Elevated diaphragm
4. Pulmonary infarction
5. Completely normal chest x-ray

Lung Scan (See Fig. 22-4)
1. If normal, excludes diagnosis of pulmonary embolus
2. However, many false positives
3. Best is comparison or
    a. Perfusion (Tc-99m of I-131 tagged albumin macroaggregates) with
    b. Ventilation (Xe-133) scan

Pulmonary Angiography (the most specific test, but invasive)
1. Indications
    a. Massive embolus with shock

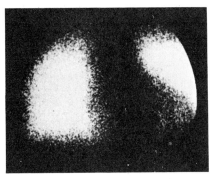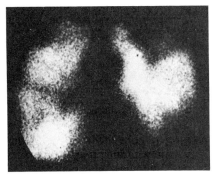

Figure 22-4 Normal radioisotope lung scan (left) and one showing multiple defects of pulmonary emboli (right).

    b. Surgical or thrombolytic therapy contemplated
    c. Anticoagulant therapy dangerous
    d. Scan not diagnostic

PATIENTS AT HIGHEST RISK

1. Hip fracture
2. Open prostatectomy
3. Patients over 40 years old
4. Pelvic operations
5. Obese
6. Previous thromboembolism
7. Neoplastic disease
8. Congestive heart failure
9. Trauma to lower extremities
10. Oral contraceptives (due to ↓ plasma Xa inhibiting factor)

ORIGIN OF EMBOLUS

1. Veins of lower extremities—75 percent
2. Pelvic veins—25 percent
3. Other—rare

THERAPY

1. Intravenous heparin: bleeding complications lower with continuous than with intermittent
2. Inferior vena caval interruption
    a. Indications
       i. Recurrent embolus while adequately anticoagulated
      ii. Anticoagulants contraindicated
     iii. Massive life-threatening embolus
    b. Methods (See Fig. 22-5)
       i. IVC ligation

240

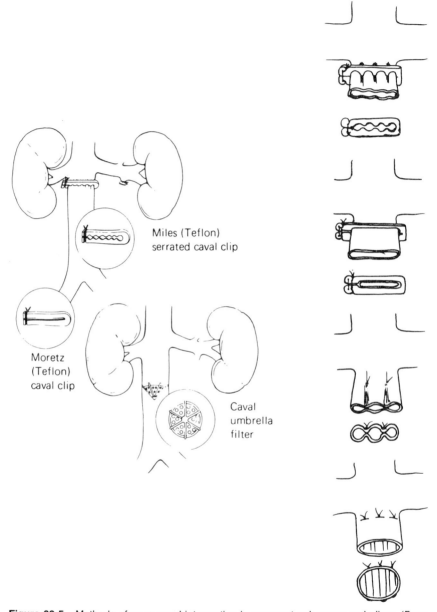

Figure 22-5 Methods of vena caval interruption in recurrent pulmonary embolism. *(From Dunphy JE and Way LW (eds):Current Surgical Diagnosis and Treatment, 3rd Edt., Lange, 1977, p 740, and Haimovici H (ed): Vascular Surgery. Principles and Techniques. McGraw-Hill, 1976, p 816, with permission.)*

        1) Tie IVC just distal to (R) renal vein
        2) (L) ovarian or testicular vein enters (L) renal vein and hence genital vein must be ligated if pelvic thrombosis exists
        3) (R) genital vein enters IVC below ligature and hence is of no concern
    ii. IVC plication
        1) Preferable to ligation because it allows recanalization
        2) Use suture compartmentalization or Adams-DeWeese clip
    iii. Mobin-Uddin or Greenfield umbrella filter
        1) Introduced from internal jugular or femoral vein cutdown under fluoroscopic control
        2) Useful especially if patient too sick for general or spinal anesthesia
        3) Complications: embolization of filter; thrombosis of IVC
  3. Pulmonary embolectomy
    a. Indications
    i. Large, life-threatening embolism
    ii. It is unusual for a patient with this problem to survive long enough for embolectomy
    iii. IVC may be tied at same time
    iv. Thrombolysin may be alternative

PROPHYLAXIS OF PULMONARY EMBOLISM

1. Rationale
    a. Two-thirds of deaths from PE occur within one-half hour
    b. 80 percent of patients die without suspicion of PE
2. Methods
    a. Mechanical (including intraoperatively)
      i. Elevation of legs
      ii. Elastic stockings
      iii. Leg exercises
      iv. Electrical calf stimulation
      v. Pneumatic compression of legs
    b. Low-dose subcutaneous heparin
      i. 5000 units s/c Q 8-12 hours starting two hours preoperatively
      ii. *Proven effective*
      iii. Mechanism: potentiates plasma inhibitor of activated factor X

SELECTED BIBLIOGRAPHY

Dale AE: The swollen leg. Curr Probl Surg, January 1973
May R: Surgery of the veins of the leg and pelvis. Major Probl Clin Surg 23:85, 1979
Silver D: Pulmonary embolism: Prevention, detection and nonoperative management. Surg Clin North Am 54:1089, 1974
Stillman RM: Venous disease. In Sawyer PN, Stillman RM: Vascular Diseases: Current Controversies. New York, Appleton-Century-Crofts, 1981, p 161

QUESTIONS

DIRECTIONS: Each of the questions or incomplete statements below is followed by five suggested answers or completions. Select the *one* that is *best* in each case.

---

1. A 48-year-old female in the intensive care unit four days after a laparotomy for ruptured spleen develops fever, chills, and a red streak from a cutdown site at the left ankle to the groin. Pus is expressed from the vein at the ankle incision. In addition to intravenous antibiotics, appropriate therapy includes:
   A. Intravenous Dextran
   B. Hot soaks and elevation
   C. Streptokinase
   D. Ligation of the greater saphenous vein at the groin
   E. Excision of the greater saphenous vein

2. The intrinsic clotting system is triggered by activation of factor:
   A. II
   B. III
   C. VI
   D. VIII
   E. XII

3. The major reason for recurrent varicose veins after stripping and ligation is:
   A. Ligation too low at saphenofemoral junction
   B. Persistent greater saphenous vein
   C. Persistent accessory saphenous vein
   D. Large perforating veins
   E. None of these

A 60-year-old female who is 48 hours post total abdominal hysterectomy complains of sudden shortness of breath and pleuritic chest pain.

4. If these complaints result from pulmonary embolism, the initial test most likely to reveal an abnormality is:
   A. Chest x-ray
   B. Electrocardiogram
   C. Complete blood count
   D. Lower extremity phlebography
   E. Arterial blood gases

5. The most common finding on chest x-ray would be:
   A. Pulmonary infiltrate
   B. Pleural effusion
   C. Elevated hemidiaphragm
   D. Pulmonary infarction
   E. No abnormal finding

6. EKG findings suggestive of pulmonary embolism include all of the following *except*:
   A. Right bundle branch block

    B. First degree heart block

    C. Acute right-axis deviation

    D. S1 pattern

    E. T3 pattern

7. The most likely site of origin of the pulmonary embolus in this patient is:

    A. Pelvic veins

    B. Veins of lower extremity

    C. Veins of upper extremity

    D. Inferior vena cava

    E. Right atrium

8. Assume that lung scan confirms pulmonary embolus in this patient. Her arterial oxygen is somewhat low, but rises to normal on nasal oxygen. She appears clinically stable and her symptoms resolve. Treatment of choice is:

    A. Low-dose subcutaneous heparin

    B. Thrombolysin and intravenous heparin

    C. Intravenous heparin

    D. Ligation of inferior vena cava and heparinization

    E. No specific therapy

9. Her partial thromboplastin time remains 2½ times control during therapy. On the fifth postoperative day, she suffers another embolus confirmed by comparison of perfusion and ventilation lung scans. Appropriate therapy now includes:

    A. Continued anticoagulation alone

    B. Ligation of inferior vena cava and left ovarian vein

    C. Ligation of inferior vena cava and right ovarian vein

    D. Ligation of inferior vena cava and both ovarian veins

    E. Pulmonary embolectomy

10. The most common biochemical elevation in pulmonary embolism is:

    A. Serum LDH

    B. Serum SGOT

    C. Serum SGPT

    D. Serum CPK

    E. Serum bilirubin

11. The most common clinical finding in pulmonary embolism is:

    A. Hemoptysis

    B. Clinically evident deep venous thrombosis

    C. Pleural friction rub

    D. Cough

    E. Tachypnea

ANSWERS

1. **E** This is *not* deep venous thrombosis; it is suppurative thrombophlebitis and should be treated as any other abscess with drainage. In this case, antibiotics and excision of the involved greater saphenous vein are indicated.

2. **E** Contact of blood with a surface other than normal intima leads to activation of the Hageman factor (XII). This leads to the cascade of factors in the intrinsic system: XI (PTA), IX (PTC), X (Stuart factor), II (prothrombin), thrombin, fibrinogen (I), fibrin. Tissue factors activate the extrinsic system by conversion of X to Xa, and then proceed as above.

3. **A** About 50 percent of recurrent varicose veins are due to a ligation performed low at the saphenofemoral junction. This causes valvular insufficiency with recurrence through tributaries in that area. The other choices are less common causes of recurrence.

4. **E** Po_2 is decreased in all cases of pulmonary embolism.

5. **A** Chest x-ray reveals pulmonary infiltrate in 57 percent of patients with symptomatic pulmonary embolism.

6. **B** First degree heart block is not a characteristic of pulmonary embolism.

7. **B** Most pulmonary emboli originate from deep veins of the lower extremity.

8. **C** Intravenous intermittent or continuous full-dose heparinization is the treatment of choice for pulmonary embolism. PTT must be kept at least 2 to 2½ times control.

9. **B** Recurrent embolism while on *adequate* heparinization is an indication for inferior vena caval interruption. In the female, ligation of the left ovarian vein is also performed since it drains into the (L) renal vein, which is above the ligature. Ligation of the testicular vein in the male may not be necessary due to its small diameter. Pulmonary embolectomy is reserved for life-threatening emboli.

10. **A** LDH rises in 83 percent of patients with PE.

11. **E** Tachypnea is most common clinical finding.

23. Pediatric Surgery

RESPIRATORY DISTRESS

1. Immediate management: Insure airway (suction), breathing, circulation
2. Aids to quick diagnosis
   a. Attempt to pass nasogastric tube down each nostril
   b. Obtain chest and abdominal x-rays
   c. Look at pharynx and larynx

Surgical Causes of Respiratory Distress

Problem	Clinical Manifestations	Diagnosis	Therapy
Choanal atresia (posterior nares)	Cyanosis when baby sleeps (mouth closed)	Inability to pass tube down nostrils	Plastic airway; dilatations
Diaphragmatic hernia (usually through pleuroperitoneal canal of Bochdalek; usually on left side)	Progressive respiratory distress as gut (now in chest) fills with air	Heart sounds shift to right; chest x-ray shows bowel in chest	Prompt reduction; repair through abdominal approach; gastrostomy may leave ventral hernia if tension in abdomen
Pneumothorax (spontaneous, traumatic, ruptured bleb, secondary to ventilatory support)	None → Severe respiratory distress	Chest x-ray	Tube thoracostomy to underwater drainage
Congenital lobar emphysema (due to partial bronchial obstruction or primary alveolar fibrosis)	Emphysematous lobe acts as a large mass, compressing normal lung and shifting mediastinum	Chest x-ray	Resection of involved lobe
Esophogeal atresia (87 percent have distal tracheo-	1. Excessive drooling 2. Aspiration,	1. Inability to pass stiff nasogastric tube	1. Gastrostomy & treatment of pneumonia;

continued

Problem	Clinical Manifestations	Diagnosis	Therapy
esophageal fistula)—failure of fusion of tracheo-esophageal septum	coughing, cyanosis when feeding 3. Vomitus contains no bile 4. Associated anomalies in 50 percent 5. Often premature	2. Esophagogram	early surgical correction via thoracotomy —may require colon interposition between 6 & 18 months of age
Cervical teratoma (superior mediastinum)	1. Airway obstruction 2. May cause dystocia	Calcium often seen on x-ray	1. Intubate 2. Prompt resection
Congenital goiter	1. Mother on thyroid suppression— high TSH, which crosses placenta 2. Airway obstruction		1. Intubate 2. Administer thyroid hormone 3. If no improvement in 5 days, do subtotal thyroidectomy
Pierre-Robin Syndrome (arrest in mandibular growth)	1. Micrognathia, relative macroglossia 2. Tongue obstructs airway		Suture or wire tongue anteriorly until growth of child alleviates problem
Massive pneumoperitoneum (usually due to ruptured greater curvature of stomach)	Respiratory distress from distended, tympanitic abdomen	Massive free intraperitoneal air on x-ray	Repair

INTESTINAL OBSTRUCTION

1. Aids to quick diagnosis
   a. Maternal hydramnios
   b. Bilious vomiting
   c. Abdominal distention
   d. Failure to pass meconium stool

Common Conditions

Condition	Diagnosis	Therapy
Duodenal obstruction	1. "Double-bubble" on x-ray 2. Often associated with mongolism	1. Atresia— duodenojejunostomy 2. Annular pancreas— duodenojejunostomy

continued

Condition	Diagnosis	Therapy
		3. Obstructing band with malrotation— divide band
Small bowel atresia (Usually results from fetal vascular occlusion)	Multiple air/fluid levels on x-ray	Resection, inject saline to insure distal patency
Imperforate anus (most common)—often associated with perineal, urethral or bladder fistula in male; perineal, fossa navicularis or vaginal fistula in female	1. Massive distention 2. Invertogram (x-ray with infant in upside down position and marker on perineum shows gap from perineum to air-filled rectum)	1. Blind pouch distal to levator (IIIa—50 percent—dissect and suture pouch to perineum) 2. Blind pouch above levator (IIIb—44 percent—preliminary diverting colostomy, definitive repair between 1½ and 2 years 3. In any case, watch for and repair associated fistula
Meconium ileus (due to deranged exocrine function, failure of enzymatic digestion, impaction of dehydrated meconium in distal ileum)	Small bowel obstruction, tenacious vomitus, masses in abdomen, sweat test for cystic fibrosis	Enemas with proteolytic enzymes, usually require laparotomy for injection of enzymes or resection
Hirschsprung's disease (absent myenteric plexus ganglia usually involving rectum only)	1. Incomplete intestinal obstruction 2. Malnutrition 3. Enterocolitis 4. Barium enema shows narrowed involved colon with proximal distention 5. Transanal biopsy of rectal muscularis shows absent myenteric ganglia	Diverting colostomy initially, later definitive correction by Swenson pullthrough, Duhamel or Soave procedure
Pyloric stenosis (Boys:girl = 4:1, hereditary)	1. Gradual obstruction within 12 weeks of life 2. Projectile vomiting without bile 3. Baby remains hungry 4. "Olive" on palpation of RUQ 5. Hypokalemic metabolic alkalosis	Hydrate, correct electrolyte abnormalities, then perform pyloromyotomy (allowing mucosa to bulge through muscle)
Intussusception (usually secondary to Meckel's diverticulum or polyp)	1. Sudden intestinal obstruction, followed by rectal blood 2. Mass on right side of abdomen	1. Gentle reduction by barium enema or operatively 2. Resect intestinal lesion if present

EXTERNAL ANATOMIC DEFECTS

Defect	Complications	Therapy
Omphalocele (failure of viscera to reduce into peritoneal cavity, leaving only thin membranous covering: occurs at base of umbilical cord)	1. Bacterial invasion 2. Rupture of sac 3. Associated malrotation 4. Omphalitis may cause extrahepatic portal vein obstruction→varices which should be treated nonoperatively as long as possible	1. Antibiotics and protect area 2. < 5 cm—reduce and close in layers 3. > 5 cm—reduce and close with mesh or use silastic silo, which is slowly rolled up like a toothpaste tube, over 6 to 10 days to return viscera to abdomen (rapid reduction → respiratory compromise & compression of inferior vena cava)
Gastroschisis (full-thickness defect of anterior abdominal wall, exposed bowel without any covering, occurs lateral to umbilical cord)	1. Chemical peritonitis due to amniotic fluid 2. Bacterial invasion 3. Segment of intestinal atresia at hernia ring	AS ABOVE
Meningocele (Meningeal sac protrudes through midline defects) Meningomyelocele (with nervous tissue in sac) occurring anywhere from apex of head (encephalocele) to coccyx	1. Associated with hydrocephalus 2. Neurologic deficit may be present, such as paraplegia or neurogenic bladder	1. Early or delayed closure to protect underlying neural tissue, prevent meningitis 2. Ventriculojugular shunt for hydrocephalus 3. Prognosis for recovery of nervous function is poor
Inguinal hernia	Incarceration or strangulation	Early repair by high ligation of sac (defect is patent processus vaginalis)
Umbilical hernia	Same	Delay treatment (unless incarcerated) until childhood because most resolve spontaneously
Sacrococcygeal teratoma (contains at least 2 germ layers) familial autosomal dominant, calcium within mass in many	10 to 20 percent malignant	Excision

JAUNDICE

Condition	Diagnosis	Therapy
Biliary atresia	Jaundice, cirrhosis, portal hypertension, ascites, liver failure	1. Confirm diagnosis by limited laparotomy, liver biopsy, cholangiogram 2. Atresia of common bile duct—Roux-en-Y choledocho- jejunostomy 3. Atresia of intrahepatic duct—Kasai hepatic portoenterostomy (prognosis poor) 4. Must differentiate from (a) physiologic jaundice of newborn (result of immature glucuronyl transferase—clears within 2 weeks); (b) neonatal hepatitis; (c) inspissated bile syndrome; (d) sepsis; (e) others
Choledochal cyst (aneurysm of common bile duct)	Kinking and cystic dilatation—obstructive jaundice, cystic mass, abdominal pain	Radical excision, or if technically difficult, choledocho-cystojejunostomy

ABDOMINAL MASS

1. Aids in diagnosis
   a. Most are renal in origin, hence, intravenous pyelogram is best study; total body opacification with double-dose contrast medium on early IVP films is helpful in identifying avascular lesions
2. Obstruction of ureters with hydronephrosis or vagina with hydrometra requires anatomical correction
3. Multicystic kidney (most common abdominal mass in neonate)
   a. Unilateral
   b. Nonfamilial
   c. Diagnosed on intravenous pyelography
   d. Treatment—removal
   e. Prognosis—excellent
4. Polycystic kidney
   a. Bilateral
   b. Inherited—autosomal dominant in adult, autosomal recessive in infant variety

    c. Pain—hematuria, mass, renal failure, hypertension, proteinuria, pyuria, hematuria

    d. Diagnosis—IVP

    e. Therapy—may require transplantation

    f. Prognosis poor

	Neuroblastoma	Wilm's tumor
Origin	Precursors of sympathetic ganglion cells in adrenal or sympathetic chain	Fetal kidney tissue
Symptoms	1. Mass—irregular, large 2. Abdominal pain, distention, vomiting, diarrhea 3. Weight loss, weakness 4. Hypertension is rare 5. Neurologic symptoms due to extension to spinal canal	1. Mass 2. Abdominal pain 3. Fever 4. Hematuria 5. Hypertension in some 6. Secondary infection
Diagnosis	1. Plain films—calcification in over 50 percent 2. IVP—displacement and deformity of kidney 3. Urinalysis—catecholamines and their breakdown products 4. Bone marrow aspiration may show metastases 5. Chest x-ray—for metastases 6. Inferior vena cavagram	1. Plain films—calcification in 10 percent 2. IVP—distortion of pelves and calices, also 6 percent will have bilateral involvement 3. Chest x-ray 4. Inferior vena cavagram 5. Cystoscopy to rule out bladder implants
Therapy	1. Large, difficult resection—biopsy then irradiate, resect later 2. Otherwise—resect, irradiate (metastases evident in 60–90 percent)	1. First ligate vessels, then perform radical excision with all involved structures and lymph nodes 2. Shell out tumor if bilateral 3. Supravoltage radiotherapy (except Stage I in infants)
Significance of Metastases	1. Liver, skin, bone marrow does *not* alter survival rate! 2. Bone—decreases survival	1. Chest (20–50 percent) but should be treatad vigorously 2. Bone—rare
Chemotherapy	Cyclophosphamide and Vincristine	Actinomycin D and Vincristine

continued

	Neuroblastoma	**Wilm's tumor**
Prognosis	1. Thoracic—90 percent survival 2. Abdominal—25 percent survival 3. Spontaneous regression has been documented in 5 percent—may be related to tumor antibodies 4. Follow urine catecholamines	1. No metastases—90 percent 2. Metastases— 40–50 percent

SELECTED BIBLIOGRAPHY

Hendren WH: Symposium on pediatric surgery. Surg Clin North Am 56:243, 1976
Ravitch MM, et al. (eds): Pediatric Surgery, 3rd Edt. Chicago, Year Book Medical
    Publishers, 1979

QUESTIONS

You are called to the delivery room to see a cyanotic premature newborn in obvious respiratory distress.
1. The first thing to do is:
    A. Start cardiac massage
    B. Intubate
    C. Perform tracheostomy
    D. Pass nasogastric tube
    E. Suction
2. The child responds well to your initial therapy. Important diagnostic tests include all *except:*
    A. Pass nasogastric tube down each nostril
    B. Obtain abdominal x-ray
    C. Perform laryngoscopy
    D. Order chest x-ray
    E. Schedule upper gastrointestinal series
3. The child is noted over the next few days to have excessive drooling, vomitus devoid of bile. Chest x-ray reveals infiltrate. The most likely diagnosis is:
    A. Congenital lobar emphysema
    B. Duodenal obstruction
    C. Esophogeal atresia with tracheoesophogeal fistula
    D. Idiopathic respiratory distress syndrome
    E. Pierre-Robin syndrome

You are called to see a month-old infant. His mother informs you that he has had increasing vomiting since birth.

4. Indications that the vomiting is due to pyloric stenosis include all of the following *except:*
   A. Bilious vomiting
   B. Hypokalemic metabolic alkalosis
   C. Failure to pass a meconium stool
   D. Palpable mass in right upper quadrant
   E. Maternal hydramnios

5. Appropriate initial treatment for this infant is:
   A. Nasogastric suction until obstruction resolves
   B. Gastrostomy
   C. Gastrojejunostomy
   D. Partial gastrectomy
   E. Pyloromyotomy

6. Appropriate treatment for a three-year-old child with his second episode of variceal bleeding and esophogeal varices is:
   A. Nonoperative
   B. Side-to-side portacaval shunt
   C. End-to-side portacaval shunt
   D. Mesocaval shunt
   E. Distal splenorenal shunt

7. The most common type of esophageal atresia includes:
   A. Blind proximal pouch, distal tracheoesophageal fistula
   B. Blind distal pouch, proximal tracheoesophageal fistula
   C. Distal and proximal tracheoesophageal fistula
   D. No tracheoesophageal fistula
   E. None of these

8. Congenital goiter usually occurs in babies whose mothers:
   A. Had untreated hyperthyroidism
   B. Had untreated hypothyroidism
   C. Received thyroid suppression
   D. Received supplemental thryoxine or T3
   E. Received radioactive iodine therapy

9. The most common cause of neonatal massive pneumoperitoneum is:
   A Perforated duodenal ulcer
   B. Perforated colon
   C. Hirshsprung's disease with enterocolitis
   D. Ruptured stomach
   E. Iatrogenic

10. The most common type of anorectal anomaly in newborns is:
    A. Type I—stenosis of terminal rectum
    B. Type II—failure of rupture of proctodeum
    C. Type III—true anal atresia
    D. Type IV—rectal atresia, normal anus ends as blind pouch

DIRECTIONS: Each group of items below consists of four or five lettered headings followed by a list of numbered words or phrases. For *each* numbered word or phrase, select the *one* lettered heading or lettered component that is most closely associated with it. Each lettered heading or lettered component may be selected once, more than once, or not at all.

A   Duodenal atresia
B   Jejunoileal atresia
C   Imperforate anus
D   Meconium ileus
E   Hirschsprung's disease

11. Rectal biopsy diagnostic
12. Double bubble on x-ray
13. Result of vascular accident
14. Associated with mucoviscidosis
15. Associated with Trisomy 21

A   Omphalocele
B   Gastroschisis
C   Meningocele
D   Meningomyelocele
E   Sacrococcygeal teratoma

16. Often calcified
17. Nervous tissue herniates
18. Chemical peritonitis always present

A   Multicystic kidney
B   Polycystic kidney
C   Neuroblastoma
D   Wilm's tumor
E   None of the above

19. Most common abdominal mass in neonate
20. Usually bilateral
21. Usually calcified

A   Neuroblastoma
B   Wilm's tumor
C   Both
D   Neither

22. Calices usually distorted on IVP
23. Spontaneous regression in 5 percent
24. Radiosensitive
25. Prognosis dismal

ANSWERS

1. E
2. E
3. C
4. A
5. E
6. A
7. A
8. C
9. D
10. C
11. E
12. A
13. B
14. D
15. A
16. E
17. D
18. B
19. A
20. B
21. C
22. B
23. A
24. C
25. D

24. Anesthesiology

REGIONAL ANESTHESIA

1. Mechanism of action and clinical correlates
   a. The axoplasm contains a high concentration of potassium and excludes sodium by a pump; hence, $-90 \mu V$ potential difference exists across this semipermeable lipoprotein membrane
   b. Stimulus to receptor → membrane becomes permeable → sodium ingress and potassium egress → propagation throughout nerve
   c. Local anesthetics alter this membrane → blockage of ion exchange in response to stimulus
   d. However, this blocking effect is best at high pH; local anesthetics' action inhibited by high pH such as in inflamed area
   e. Blocking effect is most rapid for small-diameter axons—that is, those carrying response to pinprick and temperature, not those for deep pain, position, motor, and touch
   f. The outer fibers of mixed nerves are affected first as anesthetic diffuses—these supply proximal areas, which are thus anesthetized first
   g. Recovery as the agent wears off occurs in the reverse order
2. Adverse reactions
   a. Allergic reactions—itching, urticaria, angioneurotic edema, asthma
   b. Convulsions: result from blockage of cerebral inhibitory centers → excitement, muscle twitching, seizures
   c. Unconsciousness: results from blockage of excitatory, vasomotor and respiratory centers → somnolence, coma, cardiorespiratory arrest
   d. Circulatory collapse: results from
      i. Smooth muscle relaxation → vasodilatation → hypotension
      ii. Diminished cardiac conduction
3. Safe use of regional anesthetics
   a. Take time to explain procedure to patient; beware of children and emotionally unstable patients
   b. Use minimal concentration and smallest volume
   c. Avoid intravenous injection and large topical doses (maximum for lidocaine is 500 mg)
   d. Use epinephrine (1:200,000 or 1:100,000) to decrease systemic absorption; but beware of tachycardia and cardiac arrhythmias; never use epinephrine for digital block
   e. Always have immediately available:
      i. For cardiorespiratory depression: cardiopulmonary resuscitation

    ii. For convulsions
       1) diazepam (Valium) 10 mg IV, or Pentothal 50−100 mg IV
       2) oxygen
    iii. For allergic reactions:
       1) oxygen, aminophylline 250 mg IV and
       2) diphenhydramine (Benadryl) 50 mg IV

SPINAL ANESTHESIA

1. Methods
   a. Subarachnoid
      i. Lumbar puncture between L1 and S1
      ii. For low spinal, add 10 percent Dextrose to make solution hyperbaric
      iii. For higher block, add distilled water
      iv. Add epinephrine or phenylephrine to prolong duration
   b. Epidural
      i. Needle or catheter inserted into epidural space
      ii. Avoids subarachnoid puncture, and hence post-spinal headaches
      iii. Allows very prolonged duration of effect by continuous injection of agent through catheter
2. Complications
   a. Reactions to the local agent used as detailed previously
   b. Hypotension; give fluids, Trendelenburg position, vasoconstrictors
   c. Headaches—occur in 15 percent of cases
      i. Larger caliber needles → spinal fluid leakage → headache
      ii. Usually worsens in erect position
      iii. Treatment
         1) Recumbent position
         2) Hydration
         3) Analgesics
         4) If intractable, epidural injection of 10 ml of patient's blood (plugs leak ?)
   d. Neurologic damage—rare

GENERAL ANESTHESIA

1. Commonly used agents
   a. Nitrous oxide (N_2O)
      i. Low potency—requires high concentration and supplementation with other agents → potential for hypoxia
      ii. Low solubility → fast recovery
   b. Cyclopropane (C_3H_6)
      i. Wide therapeutic/toxic margin → well tolerated by patient in shock
      ii. Releases epinephrine → increases cardiac output

   iii. Respiratory depression → hypercapnia → arrhythmias and
    hypotension ("cyclo shock")
   iv. Highly explosive
  c. Diethyl ether ($CH_3CH_2-O-CH_2CH_3$)
   i. Very wide therapeutic/toxic margin
   ii. High solubility → slow induction and recovery
   iii. Irritates respiratory passages → excessive secretions and laryngospasm
   iv. Explosive
   v. Low cost of administration—no machinery needed
  d. Halothane = Fluothane ($BrClHCCF_3$)
   i. Circulatory depressant
   ii. Smooth induction
   iii. Little respiratory irritation
   iv. Moderate muscle relaxation
   v. Hepatitis—due to breakdown product (?)
  e. Enflurane = Ethrane ($CHClFCF_2OCHF_2$)
   i. Similar to halothane
   ii. Decreased induction of arrhythmias
  f. Methoxyflurane = Penthrane ($CHCl_2CF_2OCH_3$)
   i. Dose-related high-output renal failure
  g. Ketamine (Ketalar)
   i. Parenteral (intravenous or intramuscular)
   ii. Induces trancelike state → unpleasant hallucinations during recovery
   iii. No respiratory depression, muscle relaxation, or circulatory
    depression; in fact, increases blood pressure
   iv. Short duration of anesthesia
  h. Narcotics (morphine, meperidine, fentanyl)
   i. Minimal circulatory depression
   ii. May cause significant respiratory depression
   iii. May be reversed with naloxone (Narcan)
  i. Barbiturates (thiopental, thiamylal)
   i. Used mainly for induction
   ii. Excessive doses saturate body tissues—due to slow hepatic
    metabolism, awakening may be slow
   iii. Decreases blood pressure—watch out for patients with hypovolemia or
    in shock
   iv. Inadvertant intraarterial dose → gangrene
  j. Neuromuscular blockers
   i. Tubocurarine (curare) and gallamine triethiodide (Flaxedil)
    1) Compete with acetylcholine at neuromuscular junction
    2) Antagonized by neostigmine (Prostigmin), which inhibits
     cholinesterase. However, neostigmine has muscarinic effects which
     should be blocked by atropine
   ii. Succinylcholine (Anectine), decamethonium bromide (Syncurine)
    1) Act like acetylcholine—depolarize motor end-plate membrane
    2) Hence, not easily reversed by neostigmine

3) Also, pseudocholinesterase deficiency → prolonged paralysis—treatment if this happens is prolonged mechanical ventilation

   iii. In general, neuromuscular blockers diminish required dose of general anesthetics when muscle relaxation is needed; also, they do not cross placental barrier

Systemic Effects of Commonly Used Inhalation Agents

1. Respiratory
   a. Inhibitors of mucociliary activity → retained tracheobronchial secretions → atelectasis → pneumonia
   b. Avoid by periodic "sigh" during anesthesia; inspiratory exercises (especially, incentive spirometer)
   c. Smokers, chronic lungers, obese patients, and uncooperative patients are particularly prone to these complications
   d. Hypercapnia → bronchoconstriction (halothane and ethrane are bronchodilators)
2. Circulatory
   a. Halothane, enflurane and isoflurane → decrease myocardial performance → decreased cardiac work → decreased oxygen demand → increased tolerance for hypotension and decreased coronary flow
   b. Also inhibit actomyosin ATPase → peripheral vasodilatation
   c. However, surgical stimulation in light plane of anesthesia → sympathetic stimulation → increased circulating catecholamines → tachycardia and hypertension → increased oxygen demand. This can be a problem in patients with coronary artery disease: *Postoperative myocardial reinfarction,* which carries a 50 percent mortality rate, occurs in
        i. 35 percent of patients who had myocardial infarct within 3 months of operation
        ii. 15 percent if 3 to 6 months
        iii. 5 percent if over 6 months
3. Renal
   a. Decreased urine output and increased urine/plasma osmolarity
   b. Result from
        i. Hypotension; cardiac depression
        ii. Increased antidiuretic hormone (ADH)
        iii. Catecholamines
        iv. Activation of renin–angiotensin system
   c. Rx: adequate hydration
4. Hepatic
   a. Decreased hepatic flow → decreased margin of safety to other factors affecting hepatic flow, such as:
        i. Positive pressure breathing
        ii. Surgical manipulation
        iii. Hypocarbia
   b. Halothane appears to result in hepatitis in 1/10,000 cases; however, this

may be related to high-risk operations and multiple exposures to this agent. Mechanism debated

5. Central nervous system
   a. Decreased cerebral metabolic rate → increased cerebral blood flow → increased intracranial pressure
   b. This is exacerbated by hypoxia, space-occupying lesions, cerebral edema
   c. This is lessened by alveolar hypoventilation
   d. May result in seizure patterns on EEG (especially enflurane)
6. Eyes
   a. Decreased intraocular pressure
   b. However, succinylcholine → increased intraocular pressure

Malfunctioning Equipment
1. *Unexplained hypoxia* → check
   a. Endotracheal tube (clogged? slipped out of trachea? in right main-stem bronchus?)
   b. Check for pneumothorax
   c. Check equipment (in the meantime, VENTILATE WITH BAG AND MASK)— there have been several deaths because of reversed O_2 and N_2O pipes

MALIGNANT HYPERTHERMIA (causes death in 1/20,000 anesthetized patients)

Mechanism
1. Muscle disease which appears to affect mitochondria → increased sympathetic activity → sudden release of catecholamines and thyroid hormone
2. Associated with all inhalation agents and usually triggered by succinylcholine
3. However, may occur even without anesthesia, as a result of emotional stress or physical stress and may be the cause of sudden death in athletes

Predisposing Factors
1. Hereditary—as autosomal dominant
2. Young male with musculoskeletal abnormalities including:
   a. Short stature
   b. Pectus carinatum
   c. Kyphosis or lordosis
   d. Weak serrati muscles
   e. Ptosis
   f. Antimongoloid slant of palpebral fissures
   g. Low-set ears
   h. Cryptorchidism
3. Increased serum creatine phosphokinase; this is *not* a constant finding

Clinical Findings
1. Tachycardia
2. Extreme hyperthermia; skin feels hot

3. Tachypnea if patient breathing spontaneously
4. Increased oxygen consumption → dark venous blood in operative field
5. Hyperkalemia, acidosis, shock

Therapy
1. TERMINATE SURGERY AND ANESTHESIA AS SOON AS POSSIBLE
2. Give dantrolene (Dantrium) 10 mg/kg body weight; this is a skeletal muscle relaxant
3. Cool by:
   a. Gastric or peritoneal lavage
   b. Immersion in ice water
   c. Ice packs (not very effective)
   d. Extracorporeal circulation (rarely used)
4. Hyperventilate; monitor blood gases
5. Treat hyperkalemia and acidosis
6. Give osmotic diuretic; monitor urine output
7. Use procainamide, not lidocaine, for arrhythmias

Prognosis
1. Death—60 percent
2. Late complications:
   a. Disseminated intravascular coagulopathy (DIVC)
   b. Acute tubular necrosis
   c. Irreversible coma

Prevention
1. Check patients at risk with muscle biopsy; using in vitro caffeine-halothane contracture test
2. Susceptible patients should get dantrolene prophylactically; or avoid general anesthesia if possible

OVERALL ANESTHETIC RISK

1. Overall, general anesthesia death rate is about 1 in 2000 cases
2. Risk directly related to physical status:

   Class I — no systemic problems
        II — moderate, but controlled, systemic problems
        III — severe or uncontrolled systemic problems
        IV — life-threatening systemic problems
        V — moribund
   Suffix E — emergency operation

SELECTED BIBLIOGRAPHY

Vandam LD: Anesthesia: The state of the art. Curr Probl Surg 17(7), July 1980

QUESTIONS

DIRECTIONS: Each of the questions or incomplete statements below is followed by five suggested answers or completions. Select the *one* that is *best* in each case.

1. Thirty minutes after an uneventful cholecystectomy, a 30-year-old female is noted to be restless and cyanotic. Blood pressure is 120/70, pulse 110 and, respiration is 21 per minute and shallow. The most appropriate procedure at this point is:
   A. Obtain lung scan
   B. Sedate
   C. Ventilate
   D. Start antibiotic therapy
   E. Start heparin therapy
2. A postoperative patient breathing room air has the following arterial blood gas values: $pO_2 = 60$ mmHg, $pCO_2 = 60$ mmHg, pH = 7.25. Appropriate management includes:
   A. Sedation
   B. Sodium bicarbonate
   C. Ammonium chloride
   D. Increased ventilation
   E. No specific therapy
3. Which of the following agents is associated with postoperative liver necrosis?
   A. Methoxyflurane
   B. Ether
   C. Pentothal
   D. Halothane (Fluothane)
   E. Curare
4. The maximum volume that can be expelled after a maximum inspiration without limit of time is called?
   A. Total lung capacity
   B. Inspiratory capacity
   C. Functional residual capacity
   D. Vital capacity
   E. Tidal volume
5. During suture of a facial laceration under Xylocaine local anesthesia, a 30-year-old female develops confusion, anxiety, and then convulsions. Appropriate immediate therapy is:
   A. Tracheostomy
   B. Blood transfusion
   C. Sodium Pentothal
   D. Diphenylhydantoin (Dilantin)
   E. Observation alone

6. Severe hyperkalemia in patients undergoing anesthesia for the treatment of thermal injury is most likely due to which of the following agents?
   A. Pentothal
   B. Nitrous oxide
   C. Morphine sulfate
   D. Halothane (Fluothane)
   E. Succinylcholine

7. Catecholamine-induced cardiac arrhythmias are enhanced most by the use of:
   A. Nitrous oxide
   B. Diethyl ether
   C. Cyclopropane
   D. Methoxyflurane
   E. Halothane (Fluothane)

8. The most common postoperative problem that should be anticipated in the obese patient undergoing general anesthesia is:
   A. Anesthetic accumulation in adipose tissue
   B. Anerobic metabolism
   C. Atelectasis
   D. Fat embolism
   E. Hypotension

9. The most common complication of spinal anesthesia is:
   A. Hypertension
   B. Peripheral neuropathy
   C. Headache
   D. Urinary retention
   E. Meningitis

10. The most accurate method for diagnosing hypoventilation is:
    A. Measurement of arterial pCO_2
    B. Measurement of arterial pO_2
    C. Determination of minute volume
    D. Measurement of cardiac output
    E. Clinical observation

11. Which of the following methods of ventilatory support is most likely to result in a tension pneumothorax?
    A. Pressure control ventilation
    B. Volume control ventilation
    C. Intermittent mandatory ventilation (IMV)
    D. Intermittent positive pressure ventilation
    E. Positive and expiratory pressure (PEEP) ventilation

12. Pulmonary complications in surgical patients most commonly result from:
    A. Hypercapnea
    B. Emphysema
    C. Thrombembolism
    D. Pulmonary hypertension
    E. Retained tracheobronchial secretions

13. Of the following, the most likely reason for the sudden development of bigeminy during a laparoscopic tubal ligation in an otherwise healthy 30-year-old female is:
    A. Inadequate ventilation
    B. Hypokalemia
    C. Air embolism
    D. Uncorrected blood loss
    E. Hypocalcemia

ANSWERS

1. **C** This is a typical case of prolonged duration of anesthetic effect and too early an extubation postoperatively. Typically the patient is restless with shallow respiration and may be cyanotic. Blood gases will reveal a hypoxia with a respiratory acidosis, but prompt recognition on clinical signs alone should be possible. Ventilation by bag and mask or reintubation is indicated and will be life-saving. This is a bit too early for pulmonary embolism, but if for any reason you did consider it, a lung scan would be appropriate, but only after basic life support has been initiated.

2. **D** This is a respiratory acidosis due to hypoventilation. Ventilation by bag and mask or intubation is required. Sedation is contraindicated.

3. **D** Halothane is a rare cause of postoperative jaundice and liver malfunction and hence should not be used in patients with hepatic insufficiency.

4. **D** The vital capacity is the most frequently used lung-volume measurement. It is the maximum volume that can be expelled after a maximum inspiration without limit of time and is the gross index of the ventilatory reserve in the conscious and cooperative patient. The normal range is 65 to 75 milliliters per kilogram of body weight.

5. **C** Although xylocaine (Lidocaine) local anesthesia is one of the safest drugs available, there are several complications of which one must be aware when using this drug routinely. Mild allergic reactions—urticaria, itching, angioneurotic edema, or asthma—are treated with Benadryl, oxygen, aminophylline. Circulatory depression characterized by hypotension requires the use of ephedrine sulfate, oxygen. Anxiety and convulsions are treated with sodium Pentothal 50 to 100 mg intravenously, oxygen, and adequate ventilation. Severe cardiorespiratory depression may require cardiopulmonary support.

6. **E** A number of patients undergoing anesthesia for the treatment of burns and patients with muscle trauma or neurologic problems have developed severe hyperkalemia, even to the point of cardiac arrest, which appears to be related to increased sensitivity of the muscle membrane to succinylcholine.

7. **C** Cyclopropane tends to increase cardiac output and arterial pressure due to sympathetic stimulation and vasoconstriction. It also sensitizes the

heart to catecholamines, with a resultant tendency to dangerous arrhythmias.

8. **C** During anesthesia the obese patient has reduced tidal volume due to elevation of the diaphragm and often poor inspiratory efforts. This will lead to atelectasis and should be prevented with encouragement of coughing and deep breathing before and after surgery.

9. **C** The use of a small-gauge needle and having the patient remain supine for 12 hours lessens the incidence of post-spinal anesthesia headache.

10. **A** The best measurement of the adequacy of ventilation is the arterial carbon dioxide tension. The arterial oxygen concentration can be easily influenced by impaired alveolar capillary diffusion. The patient's respiratory rate, tidal volume, or minute volume do not in themselves determine the adequacy of a patient's ventilation.

11. **E** Positive and expiratory pressure can prevent alveolar collapse at the end of expiration by maintaining a small positive pressure. This is most useful in treatment of the adult respiratory distress syndrome, in which hypoxia persists despite increasing inspired oxygen concentration. It does have its complications, however. These include decreased cardiac output and pneumothorax.

12. **E** A patient developing fever within the first 24 to 48 hours after surgery under general anesthesia most likely has atelectasis and retained tracheobronchial secretions. The conscious person will periodically sigh—that is, take a deep breath—to expand the lung fully and cough to expel secretions. This often is not the case with anesthetized patients. This is the reason patients are encouraged to cough, deep breathe, and often use incentive spirometers postoperatively.

13. **A** When cardiac arrhythmias occur in an anesthetized or early postoperative patient who is otherwise healthy, always consider ventilation first. In this case, the endotracheal tube may have inadvertently passed into the esophagus, may be occluded, or mechanical ventilation may be insufficient. Although blood loss and electrolyte abnormalities may cause cardiac arrhythmias also, they are unlikely in this case.

25. Skin and Soft Tissue

MELANOMA

1. *Etiology:* chronic irritation from sunlight, trauma, elastic bands of clothing, radiation
2. *Location: anywhere*
3. *Appearance:* one-quarter arise from preexistant nevus with change in size, appearance, seepage of serum, bleeding, nodule formation, ulceration, satellite lesion formation

Clinical Classification
1. Lentigo maligna (Hutchinson's melanotic freckle): best prognosis, occurs in sun-exposed areas of malar and temporal regions
2. Superficial spreading melanoma: intermediate prognosis
3. Nodular melanoma: worst prognosis; melanoma without adjacent intraepidermal component

Histologic Classification (Clark's)

Class	Description	Chance of Nodal Metastases	Mortality
I	All tumor cells superficial to basement membrane	0%	0%
II	Into loose connective tissue of papillary dermis	4	8
III	Junction of papillary and reticular dermis	7	35
IV	Into reticular dermis	49	46
V	Into subcutaneous tissue	70	55

Clinical Correlates
1. Spontaneous regression of primary lesion may result in metastases without demonstrable source
2. In some cases, single pulmonary metastatic lesions may be resected and improve prognosis
3. Estrogens and pregnancy lower survival rates
4. May be confused clinically with blue nevus, a benign condition
5. Early lymphatic metastases common; later hematogenous metastases to liver, spleen, bones, brain, small bowel, breast

Treatment
1. Wide local excision or amputation (for example, for subungual lesion)
2. Regional lymph node dissection if clinically positive nodes or Clark's level IV or V. Controversial with level III
3. Perfusion of extremity with chemotherapeutic agent
4. Immunotherapy using BCG, levamisole, or patient's own melanoma cells

SOFT TISSUE TUMORS OF EXTREMITY

Work-up
1. X-ray—for local bone involvement
2. CT scan—extent of tumor, presence of tumor, nature of tumor (solid or cystic)
3. Chest x-ray—for pulmonary metastases (obtain tomograms if suspicious)
4. Angiography—for vascular involvement
5. *Incisional biopsy*—the most important and definitive test

Clinicopathologic Correlates
1. Pseudocapsule—nests and projections of sarcoma cells into surrounding tissue—DO NOT ENUCLEATE; USE INCISIONAL BIOPSY
2. Skip areas—may not be evident on examination—AVOID LIMITED EXCISIONS
3. Necrosis and hemorrhage (because tumor outgrows blood supply)—AVOID NEEDLE BIOPSY; spillage may seed tumor
4. Frozen section inaccurate—await paraffin section result before ablative therapy when possible
5. Degree of differentiation is related to survival

Treatment

Surgical excision with en-bloc removal of
1. Biopsy scar and tracts (hence, biopsy incision must be carefully planned)
2. One fascial layer (if possible)
3. All contiguous structures
4. All of the above, *without* exposure of the tumor at any time

Amputation only when
1. Adequate resection will render extremity functionless
2. No reconstructive or rehabilitative procedures will increase function
3. No alternative therapy will control systemic and local disease

Note: Local recurrence rates may be lowered by amputation, but overall survival *not* improved

Lymph node dissection
1. If clinically suspicious, biopsy nodes
2. If pathologically positive, perform node dissection
3. Palliative node dissection *not* proven beneficial

SOFT TISSUE SARCOMAS

Classification

T0 = no demonstrable tumor N0 = nodes negative M0 = No known metastases
T1 = < 5 cm N1 = nodes positive M1 = Proven metastases
(80 percent will be
pulmonary)

T2 = > 5 cm
T3 = Invades bone, major
vessel or nerve

Prognosis (in decreasing order of survival)
1. Liposarcoma 55 percent
2. Fibrosarcoma
3. Malignant fibrous histiocytoma
4. Malignant schwannoma
5. Synovial sarcoma
6. Leiomyosarcoma
7. Angiosarcoma
8. Rhabdomyosarcoma 23 percent

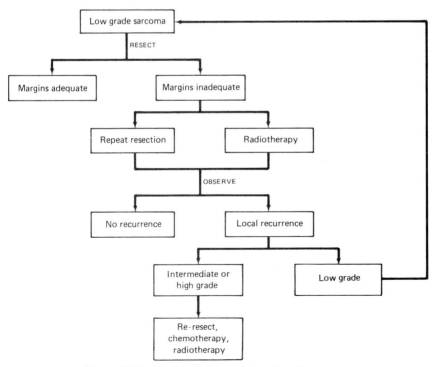

Figure 25-1 Treatment of low-grade extremity sarcoma.

9. Kaposi's sarcoma—increasing incidence with AIDS (acquired immunodeficiency syndrome) epidemic

Adjuvant Therapy (See Figure 25-1)
1. Radiation: myxoid liposarcoma and embryonal rhabdomyosarcoma are radiosensitive; others unpredictable
2. Chemotherapy: Adriamycin, Vincristine, regional perfusion
3. Palliation: is best by surgical resection, when possible

SELECTED BIBLIOGRAPHY

Kopf AW, et al.: Malignant Melanoma. New York, Masson, 1979
Shiu MH: Soft tissue sarcomas. In Alfonso AE, Gardner B: Practice of Cancer Surgery. New York, Appleton-Century-Crofts, 1982, p 293

QUESTIONS

DIRECTIONS: Each of the questions or incomplete statements below is followed by five suggested answers or completions. Select the *one* that is *best* in each case.

A 40-year-old female presents with recent ulceration of a plantar mole. Aside from this lesion, which she has had since childhood, she has been in good health.

1. The most appropriate initial approach to therapy is:
   A. Biopsy
   B. 5-FU topically
   C. Close observation
   D. Radiotherapy
   E. None of these
2. This is found to be a Clark's level II melanoma. Adequate definitive therapy is:
   A. Wide local excision alone
   B. Wide local excision with node dissection if nodes clinically positive
   C. Wide local excision with node dissection even if nodes clinically negative
   D. Amputation of foot and node dissection
   E. Amputation of leg and node dissection
3. The patient does well until six months later, when she returns with intestinal obstruction. The most likely cause is:
   A. Intussusception
   B. Adhesions
   C. Volvulus
   D. Hepatic metastases
   E. Cancer of the colon

ANSWERS

1. **A**
2. **B**
3. **A**

26. Kidneys

KIDNEY TRANSPLANTATION

CLASSIFICATION

1. Heterotransplant = xenograft = between species
2. Homotransplant = allograft = within a species
3. Autotransplant = autograft = within an individual

INDICATIONS

1. End-stage renal failure in
   a. Glomerulonephritis
   b. Pyelonephritis
   c. Polycystic kidney disease
   d. Malignant hypertension
   e. Etc.

SELECTION OF DONOR

1. ABO blood group *compatibility*—essential
2. MLC
   a. Mix donor lymphocytes, recipient lymphocytes, and tritiated thymidine
   b. Incompatible cells stimulate each other to form blasts and antibodies. This is reflected in thymidine uptake
   c. Donor cells may first be rendered nonresponsive but still antigenic using a cytotoxic agent
3. HL-A typing
   a. Method
      i. HL-A antigens are glycoproteins present in serum, saliva, and on the surfaces of all cells
      ii. They are determined in man by five loci on the sixth chromosome—A, B, C, D, DR
      iii. Present methods allow routine determination of only A and B antigens by serologic typing
      iv. Hence, each patient has potentially four antigens (two from each parent—A and B) out of a total of 30 known antigens

v. In some cases, fewer than four can be identified by available methods
   b. Significance
      i. Nonidentical siblings have a 25 percent chance of sharing all four antigens, 50 percent chance of sharing only two, and 25 percent chance of sharing none. Graft survival best with identical match in siblings
      ii. Significance in unrelated donors is controversial

TECHNIQUE (See Fig. 26-1)

Donor Operation
1. Living—(L) kidney preferable because
   a. Longest renal vein
   b. Renal artery well separated from vena cava
   c. Subcostal retroperitoneal approach is used
   d. Mortality rate 0.1 percent
2. Cadaver
   a. Pretreatment of cadaver with immunosuppressive agents appears to

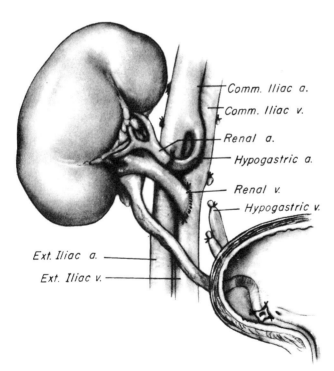

Figure 26-1 Technique of renal transplantation. *(From Schwartz SI (ed):* Principles of Surgery, *McGraw-Hill, 1969, p. 297, with permission.)*

decrease rejection by interfering with "passenger leukocytes," which are trapped within the graft and cause immune response in recipient
b. Preservation by pulsatile perfusion allows time for transportation of kidney, evaluation of compatibilities, and is possibly better for kidney than simple hypothermia

Recipient Operation
1. Usually transplant into (R) iliac fossa
2. Renal artery end-to-end of hypogastric artery
3. Renal vein end-to-side of common iliac vein
4. Ureter implanted into bladder
5. Preliminary bilateral nephrectomy indicated only if infected, or causing uncontrolled hypertension

POSTOPERATIVE THERAPY

Drugs
1. Azathioprine (Imuran)
   a. Derivative of 6-mercaptopurine
   b. Inhibits nucleic acid synthesis
   c. 2 to 3 mg/kg daily indefinitely
   d. Watch for leukopenia or thrombocytopenia
2. Prednisone
   a. 120 mg daily for three days, then reduce by 20 mg every three days
   b. Eventually may be reduced to 10 mg daily
   c. Alternate-day therapy may help reduce unwanted side effects, especially growth retardation in children
3. Antithymocyte globulin: Usually from horse sensitized to human lymphocytes; currently under study in treatment of rejection

Splenectomy, Thymectomy, Thoracic Duct Drainage, X-ray Therapy
1. Not of proven value

OTHER FACTORS IN REJECTION

1. Cadaveric graft followed by living related graft has better prognosis than the reverse
2. Multiple blood transfusions prior to transplant are protective; mechanism controversial
3. Graft survival is higher in blood type O recipients

COMPLICATIONS

Table 1. Types of Rejection

Type	Etiology	Timing	Findings	Therapy
1. Hyper-acute	Preformed cytotoxic antibodies against donor lymphocytes or renal cells	Immediately on operating table	Blue, soft kidney, renal cortical necrosis on biopsy, sudden decrease of blood flow	NONE, irreversible, must remove kidney
2. Accelerated	Subliminal preformed cytotoxic antibodies against donor cells, or sensitized cells	Within 5 days	Fever, enlarged, tender graft (due to peritoneum stretching), then oliguria, hypertension, weight gain, increased BUN, creatinine, decreased GFR, decreased urinary sodium	Increase steroids, but usually not reversible
3. Acute	Immune cellular reaction (T-cells) against foreign antigens	1–8 weeks	As above	Increase steroids, usually reversible
4. Chronic	Humoral factors	Late	Slowly decreasing renal function, proteinuria, hypertension	Increase steroids, usually not completely reversible

1. Rejection (See Table 1)
2. Acute tubular necrosis
   a. Incidence
      i. Rarely in living related
      ii. Most common cause of early oliguria in cadaveric
   b. Diagnosis
      i. Assure adequate blood volume
      ii. Assure patent Foley catheter

        iii. Increased urinary sodium excretion
        iv. IVP to rule out obstructive uropathy
        v. Renal scan (I-131 hippuran)
        vi. Needle biopsy of kidney
    c. Treatment
        i. Observation
        ii. Hemodialysis
3. Sepsis
    a. Incidence: most common cause of death in transplantation
    b. Prevention: Avoid overuse of steroids in the treatment of rejection. Sacrifice the kidney instead of the patient. Besides, recent data indicate that low-dose immunosuppression, even in rejection, does not change graft survival
    c. Organisms
        i. Usually Gram-negative or fungal
        ii. Rare organisms may cause overwhelming infection: *Pneumocystis carinii*, Cryptococcus, many others reported
    d. Treatment
        i. Stop immunotherapy
        ii. Appropriate antibiotics
4. Technical complications
    a. Lymphocele: watch for lymphatics in transplanted kidney
    b. Ureteral necrosis or leakage: blood supply to ureter is longitudinal from renal artery; hence, do not skeletonize ureter or dissect into pelvis during nephrectomy
    c. Hematoma, etc.
5. Systemic complications
    a. Complications of steroids: cataracts, Cushing's syndrome, pathologic fractures, aseptic necrosis, peptic ulcer disease, etc.
    b. Tertiary hyperparathyroidism: may require parathyroidectomy
    c. Renal artery stenosis: heralded by uncontrolled hypertension; may require operative repair
    d. Glomerulonephritis: this complication is why even identical twin transplant recipients require immunosuppression
    e. Cancer
        i. Squamous or basal cell—33 percent
        ii. Reticulum cell sarcoma—13 percent
        iii. A variety of others reported
    f. Atherosclerotic heart disease: this, however, is lessened in transplanted patients over patients on chronic hemodialysis

PROGNOSIS (improving)

1. Graft survival at two years
    a. Living-related
        i. HL-A identical—100 percent

ii. HL-A nonidentical—91 percent
  b. Cadaveric—50 percent
  c. Poorer in children and diabetics
2. Patient survival at two years
  a. Living related donors—100 percent
  b. Cadaveric donors—86 percent

RENOVASCULAR HYPERTENSION

PHYSIOLOGY

Renin
1. In kidney
  a. Produced by juxtaglomerular apparatus
  b. Released into renal veins
2. In plasma: acts on renin-substrate to produce Angiotensin I (decapeptide)
3. In lung: converting enzyme converts Angiotensin I to Angiotensin II (octapeptide)

Angiotensin II
1. Very potent direct pressor substance that constricts smooth muscle of arterioles
2. Indirectly stimulates aldosterone secretion from adrenal cortex, which causes salt and water retention

Angiotensin III (heptapeptide)
1. Less potent direct pressor substance
2. Currently under investigation

EXPERIMENTAL MODELS

One-Kidney (Volume-Dependent) Hypertension
1. Model: unilateral nephrectomy and clamp contralateral renal artery
2. Mechanism
  a. Increased renin production in clamped side →
  b. Increased adrenal aldosterone production →
  c. Increased salt and water retention (cannot be excreted by opposite kidney) →
  d. Renin shut off

3. Hence: volume-dependent hypertension with normal plasma renin-angiotensin
4. Represents clinically
   a. Bilateral renal artery stenosis   c. Reduced renal mass
   b. Renoprival hypertension   d. Uremia
5. Treatment: salt and water restriction alone

Two-Kidney (Renin-Dependent) Hypertension

1. Model: clamp one renal artery
2. Mechanism
   a. Increased renin secretion in clamped side →
   b. Increased adrenal aldosterone production →
   c. Initial salt and water retention →
   d. Excreted by opposite kidney
3. Hence: hypertension with normal salt and water balance (renin-dependent)
4. Represents clinically: unilateral renal artery stenosis
5. Treatment: correction of renal artery occlusion or nephrectomy

ETIOLOGY OF HYPERTENSION (OVERALL)

1. Essential
2. Renovascular
   a. Atherosclerotic
   b. Fibromuscular dysplasia
3. Parenchymal kidney disease
4. Other
   a. Coarctation of the aorta   c. Primary hyperaldosteronism
   b. Cushing's syndrome   d. Pheochromocytoma

ETIOLOGY OF RENOVASCULAR HYPERTENSION

	Atherosclerosis		Fibromuscular dysplasia
Incidence	2	:	1
Sex predominance	M		F
Age group	Old		Young
Location	Orifice and prox. 1/3		Middle & distal 1/3
Usual side involved	L		R

DIAGNOSIS

Screening Studies

1. History, physical, CBC, urinalysis, electrolytes, BUN, creatinine, abdominal or flank bruit
2. Urinary catecholamine levels (for pheochromocytoma)

3. Urinary adrenal steroid level, serum cortisol (for Cushing's syndrome)
4. Rapid sequence IVP (for renal parynchymal disease, renal artery stenosis, etc.)
5. Renal scan (unreliable)

Further Studies
1. Indications (debated)
   a. Diastolic over 100, and
   b. Operative candidate
2. Procedures
   a. Renal arteriography; AP *and* oblique views necessary for full visualization
   b. Differential renal vein renin studies
      i. Requires preparation with
         1) Sodium depletion (restriction and diuretics)
         2) Stop antihypertensives for two weeks (especially propranolol and Aldomet); if necessary, use guanethidine, which does not block renin
         3) Hydralazine may stimulate renin production from ischemic kidney
      ii. Interpretation
         1) Ratio of one side to the other over 1.4 is positive
         2) In borderline cases, renal:systemic renin ratios may help
   c. Split renal function studies
      i. High morbidity
      ii. Generally outdated

TREATMENT

Medical
1. If risk of surgery is high

Surgical
1. Indications—debated
2. Procedures
   a. Aortorenal bypass
      i. With autogenous saphenous vein
      ii. With autogenous hypogastric artery (if vein not available)
      iii. With prosthetic graft material
   b. Thromboendarterectomy with patch graft
   c. Ex vivo reconstruction ("Bench surgery")—Used in severe disease where complex reconstruction is contemplated
   d. Nephrectomy: last resort and hazardous due to progression of disease in contralateral kidney.

Complications
1. Persistent hypertension (more common in cases with generalized atherosclerosis)

2. Congestive heart failure and pulmonary edema postoperatively (watch daily weights and CVP)
3. Acute tubular necrosis
4. Graft problems
    i. Dilatation or aneurysm
    ii. Thrombosis (less if end-to-end)
    iii. Stenosis

SELECTED BIBLIOGRAPHY

Chatterjee SN: Organ transplantation. Surg Clin North Am 58(2): April 1978

Kaufman JJ: Symposium on the management of renovascular hypertension. Urol Clin North Am 2:215, 1975

Libertino JA, Zimman L: Technique of renal transplantation. Surg Clin North Am 53(2):455, 1973

QUESTIONS

DIRECTIONS: Each of the questions or incomplete statements below is followed by five suggested answers or completions. Select the *one* that is *best* in each case.

A 23-year-old female two days after cadaveric renal transplant develops oliguria.
1. The least likely cause of this complication is:
    A. Accelerated rejection
    B. Obstructed Foley catheter
    C. Hypovolemia
    D. Hyperacute rejection
    E. Acute tubular necrosis
2. Each of the following findings would favor rejection over acute tubular necrosis *except:*
    A. Tender graft
    B. Increased urinary sodium excretion
    C. Fever
    D. Lack of response to volume load
    E. Englarged graft
3. The likelihood of two brothers being HL-A identical in all four A and B antigens is:
    A. 25 percent
    B. 50 percent
    C. 75 percent
    D. 33 percent
    E. 100 percent

4. The most common cancer occurring in long-term transplant survivors involves the:
   A. Lymph nodes
   B. Blood
   C. Skin
   D. Colon
   E. Kidney
5. A congenital metabolic disease correctable by renal allografting is:
   A. Osler-Weber-Rendu syndrome
   B. Gaucher's disease
   C. Fabry's disease
   D. Phenylketonuria
   E. Felty's syndrome

DIRECTIONS: The group of items below consists of five lettered headings, followed by a list of numbered words or phrases. For *each* numbered word or phrase, select the *one* lettered heading or lettered component that is most closely associated with it. Each lettered heading or lettered component may be selected once, more than once, or not at all.

   A   Passenger leukocytes
   B   Plasma cells
   C   Enhancing antibody
   D   Immune lymphoid cell
   E   Blocking antibody

---

6. Responsible for antibody production
7. Responsible for acute rejection
8. Decreases destructive effect of immune cellular reaction
9. Major reason for immunosuppressive pretreatment of cadaveric donors

---

DIRECTIONS: For each of the questions or incomplete statements below, *one* or *more* of the answers or completions given is correct. Select:

   A   if only 1, 2, *and* 3 are correct
   B   if only 1 *and* 3 are correct
   C   if only 2 *and* 4 are correct
   D   if only 4 is correct
   E   if all are correct

---

10. Renal allograft survival is higher:
    1. After multiple blood transfusions
    2. In Type O recipients
    3. If living related graft follows cadaveric graft
    4. In diabetic recipients
11. Renal transplants between identical twins:
    1. Are always HL-A identical

    2. Have relatively good prognosis for long-term function

    3. Are always ABO compatible

    4. Rarely require immunosuppression

12. T cells are:
    1. Responsible for cellular immunity
    2. Present in thoracic duct lymph
    3. Responsible for delayed hypersensitivity reactions
    4. Present in normal lymph nodes

13. Azathioprine (Imuran):
    1. Inhibits nucleic acid synthesis
    2. Inhibits humoral immunity
    3. Inhibits cellular immunity
    4. Is an antimetabolite

14. Hyperacute rejection of a kidney transplant:
    1. Requires vigorous steroid therapy
    2. Is preventable by assuring negative leukocyte crossmatch
    3. Is usually reversible
    4. Is related to preformed cytotoxic antibodies

15. B cells are:
    1. Responsible for cellular immunity
    2. Present in normal lymph nodes
    3. Responsible for delayed hypersensitivity reactions
    4. Present in thoracic duct lymph

DIRECTIONS: Each of the questions or incomplete statements below is followed by five suggested answers or completions. Select the *one* that is *best* in each case.

---

16. The most common presenting finding in a patient with unilateral renal artery stenosis is:
    A. Hypertension
    B. Glomerular fibrosis
    C. Peripheral edema
    D. Hematuria
    E. Elevated blood urea nitrogen

17. Most reliable in differentiating renovascular from essential hypertension is:
    A. Renal scan
    B. Abdominal or flank bruit
    C. Rapid sequence IVP
    D. Differential renal vein renin assay
    E. Split renal function studies

18. The most reliable in predicting response to surgical therapy for renovascular hypertension:
    A. Extent of generalized atherosclerosis
    B. Creatinine level
    C. Split renal function studies

D. Uptake on renal scan
E. Renal biopsy

ANSWERS

1. **D** Hyperacute rejection occurs on the operating table. Rejection occurring after two days is most likely accelerated rejection. Other possibilities, such as hypovolemia, obstruction, or acute tubular necrosis, must be ruled out before steroids are increased in the treatment of suspected rejection.
2. **B** Rejection is characterized, among other things, by decreased urinary sodium, while ATN results usually in increased urinary sodium excretion.
3. **A** Each parent will donate one antigen for the A locus and one antigen for the B locus. The chances that two brothers have identical antigens in both these loci are one-quarter = 25 percent. Remember that both loci are on the same chromosome.
4. **C** The most common cancer found in long-term transplant recipients is squamous cell or basal cell cancer of the skin.
5. **C** Fabry's syndrome is a sex-linked error of glycosphingolipid metabolism causing deposition of trihexosyl ceramide in various sites including the kidney. This results in renal failure. Transplantation of a normal kidney provides the missing enzyme—ceramide trihexosidase.
6. **B** Plasma cells are responsible for antibody production.
7. **D** The immune lymphoid cell (T cell) causes acute rejection.
8. **E**
9. **A** Passenger leukocytes are cells trapped within a donor kidney which may elicit a severe immune response in the host.
10. **A** Diabetic recipients have a poorer renal allograft survival than the general population, but transplantation is still indicated, especially since it decreases the systemic complications of diabetes in many cases.
11. **A** Identical twins require immunosuppression to prevent the development of glomerulonephritis in the transplanted kidney.
12. **E** All these are properties of T cells.
13. **E** All are properties of azathioprine.
14. **C** Hyperacute immune rejection is due to preformed cytotoxic antibodies, which can be detected by the leukocyte crossmatch. It is not reversible and requires nephrectomy, not steroids.
15. **D** B cells are present in thoracic duct lymph and are responsible for antibody production.
16. **A** Due to increased renin production and arteriolar vasoconstriction.
17. **D** All studies have false positives and false negatives. Hence, this diagnosis is most difficult, but in the face of arteriogram demonstrating significant renal artery stenosis, differential renal vein renin assays are best in demonstrating renovascular hypertension.
18. **A** Patients with generalized ASPVD in general do poorly.

27. Wound Healing and Infection

WOUND HEALING

CLASSIFICATION AND MECHANISMS

1. First intention: clean wound, closed primarily will heal as follows:

Phase Time period	Mechanism	Clinical correlates
I. First four days	INFLAMMATION: blood exposed to collagen: a. Activates Hageman factor → kinin and complement cascade, plasmin generation, clotting mechanism b. Platelet degranulation → substances which amplify above + mitogen for fibroblasts. Also, fibrin split products attract other inflammatory cells, especially monocytes	Metabolic demand increased by active cells, while circulation decreased by capillary thrombosis → local lactic acidosis. This is increased with more dead space or tissue damage because of limited oxygen diffusion. Steriods inhibit transition to next phase
II. Up to 10th day	PROLIFERATION of a. Fibroblasts → collagen synthesis (stimulated by lactate ?) → wound develops tensile strength b. New vessels which start as capillary buds in venules	a. Collagen synthesis requires iron, oxygen, vitamin C and alphaketogluterate b. Palpation of an indurated area around the wound ("healing ridge") by the tenth day signals normal phase II healing
III. Up to 1 year	MATURATION: remodeling of collagen; by the third week collagen lysis exceeds synthesis	a. Requires collagenase b. While "healing ridge" disappears, net tensile strength increases; but never reaches strength of unwounded tissue

2. Second intention:
   a. Wound left open → granulation tissue (blood vessels, inflammatory cells,

fibroblasts, and collagen) fills dead space → epithelial cell migration covers defect
   b. Contraction: normal surrounding tissue moves into open area to fill large defects; depends on myofibroblasts; inhibited by steriods
3. Third intention (delayed primary closure):
   a. Contaminated wound left open during phase I, then closed
   b. Drainage and exposure to air for several days → decreased bacterial colonization
   c. Polymorphonuclear leukocytes and extracellular fluid opsonins kill bacteria, especially Staphylococci; membrane-bound oxidase → reduction of oxygen to superoxide → dismutation to hydrogen peroxide → conversion to microbicidal compounds

Factors Which Inhibit Healing ("DIDN'T HEAL"): ◄

1. Drugs: steroids, antimetabolites
2. Infection
3. Diabetes, uncontrolled
4. Nutrition inadequate (calories, protein, vitamins, minerals)
5. Tissue necrosis; ischemia, radiation injury
6. Hypoxia, systemic; hypovolemia
7. Excessive tension on wound edges
8. Another wound: competition among several healing areas for required substrates
9. Low temperature: extremity wounds heal relatively slowly

SURGICAL INFECTIONS

ANTIBIOTICS

For Gram-Positives
1. *Streptococcus*
   a. A-beta hemolytic—pen, erythro
   b. B-beta hemolytic (gynecologic)—pen, erythro
   c. C *(viridans)* (SBE)—pen, cephalo, vanco
   d. D *(enterococci)* (GU and SBE)—amp, pen, genta, kana
2. *Diplococcus pneumoniae*—pen (always sensitive), erythro
3. *Staphylococcus aureus*—methi, clinda

For Gram-Negatives
1. *Escherichia coli:* genta, kana, cephalo
2. *Enterobacter, Serratia* (third day surgical fever):genta, kana
3. *Klebsiella:* genta, kana, cephalo

4. *Proteus:* pen, amp
5. *Indole* (+) *proteus:* carben, genta, kana
6. *Provendentia:* carben, genta, kana
7. *Pseudomonas* (water bacteria): carben + genta, tobra

Anaerobes
1. Collect in airtight syringe; use low redox medium
2. Anaerobic streptococci (gangrene, cellulitis): pen
3. *Bacteroides fragilis* (fecalent odor, often mixed infection): clinda, chloro

COMPLICATIONS OF ANTIBIOTICS

1. Penicillin
   a. Allergic reactions
      i. 5 to 10 percent incidence
      ii. Most common from topical administration
      iii. Anaphylaxis 0.1 percent of this group
   b. Coombs' (+) hemolytic anemia
   c. Myoclonic seizures (large doses)
   d. Interstitial nephritis
2. Carbenicillin: 4.7 mEq sodium/g (and must use 30 to 40 g daily)
3. Cephalosporins
   a. Uncommon cross reaction in pen allergic individuals
   b. False-positive urine glucose tests
4. Tetracycline: hepatic necrosis if greater than 2 g daily
5. Chloramphenicol
   a. Aplastic anemia (1/30,000 patients)
   b. Use in infections resistant to other antibiotics
▶ 6. Aminoglycosides: *Kanamycin, Neomycin, Gentamycin, Streptomycin* (KiNGS)
   a. Nephrotoxicity: dose must be adjusted if creatinine is increased
7. Kanamycin: above + respiratory arrest with intraperitoneal administration
8. Clindamycin: severe colitis
9. Polymixin, colistin: nephrotoxicity

BROAD-SPECTRUM PROPHYLACTIC ANTIBIOTICS

Indications
1. Serious operations with high risk of contamination
2. Host resistance low
3. Prosthetic material, vascular suture line, or in any case where infection would be a grave complication
4. Where bronchial tree, GI, or GU tract transected

Problems
1. Proliferation of resistant organisms
2. *Must* start preoperatively to be effective

Agent: usually cephalosporin

POTENTIALLY FATAL SEPSIS OF UNKNOWN ORGANISMS

"Shotgun Therapy"
1. Clindamycin 600 mg Q6 to 8 hours, *and*
2. Penicillin 6 to 8 million units daily, *and*
3. Tobramycin or gentamycin 60 to 80 mg Q8 hours (if renal function normal)

WOUND INFECTION

Etiology
1. Over 7,500,000 Staphylococci must be inoculated into experimental wound to produce infection in normal humans
2. Usually caused by break in technique, symptomatic carrier in operating room, or transected viscus
3. Local factors
   a. Devitalized tissue
   b. Foreign body
4. Systemic factors
   a. Age
   b. Obesity
   c. Steroids
   d. Immunosuppression
   e. Immunologic disorder
   f. Diabetes
   g. Duration of operation
   h. Duration of preoperative hospitalization

Organisms
1. Coagulase-negative Staphylococcus—most frequently *cultured* from incision
2. Coagulase-positive Staphylococcus—most like to cause wound *infection*

Prevention (reduce etiologic factors)
1. Prophylactic antibiotics where indicated
2. Adherent surgical drapes (conflicting evidence)–may actually ↑ infection rate
3. For wounds prone to infection, use delayed closure (close at >4 days with Steristrips or preplaced sutures)
4. Avoid braided suture material which has interstices where bacteria can thrive

5. If possible, avoid sutures in the relatively avascular subcutaneous space
→ use subcuticular skin closure, tapes, or staples
6. Antibiotic irrigation (kanamycin)
7. Change gloves during procedure (25 percent become perforated each hour)
8. Preoperative hexachlorophene shower
9. Depilatory preparation (instead of razor); or shave on OR table, *not* night
before surgery
10. Drains should be brought out from separate incisions
11. Short preoperative hospital stay
12. Meticulous surgical technique, efficient operation

INTRAABDOMINAL ABSCESS (See Fig. 27-1)

Etiology
1. Primary (no cause found)—only 10 percent
2. Sequel of peritonitis
3. Diseased organ
4. Postoperative complication (in 1 to 2 percent of operations)

Clinical Findings
1. Change in progress of recovery
2. Pain, fever, mass, jaundice
3. Sepsis

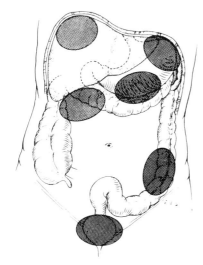

Figure 27-1 Common locations of peritoneal abscess formation. *(From Dunphy JE and Way LW (eds):* Current Surgical Diagnosis and Treatment, *3rd Edt. Lange, 1977, p 454, with permission.)*

Diagnosis by X-ray Studies

1. Pleural effusion in subphrenic abscess
2. Immobile diaphragms
3. Air/fluid level in abscess cavity
4. Lung-liver scan
5. Gallium-67 scan (but accumulates also in neoplasms, fresh incisions, and by excretion into intestine)
6. Displacement of viscus
7. Sonogram or CT scan

Therapy

1. Subphrenic
   a. Extraperitoneal approach anteriorly, or
   b. Posteriorly through transpleural route
2. Subhepatic
   a. Subcostal approach, or
   b. Posteriorly through bed of 12th rib
3. Pelvic (See Fig. 27-2)
   a. Through anterior walls of rectum, or
   b. Through posterior vaginal vault, or

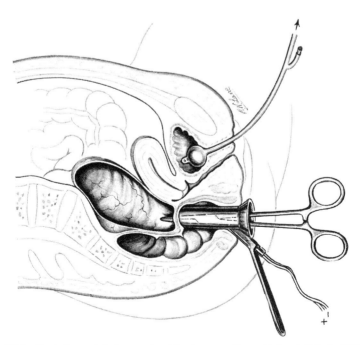

Figure 27-2 Technique of drainage of pelvic abscess. *(From Maingot R (ed):* Abdominal Operations, *6th Edt. Appleton-Century-Crofts, 1974, p 1386, with permission.)*

c. Suprapubic route (if large)
4. In selected cases, percutaneous drainage under fluoroscopic or CT control

SELECTED BIBLIOGRAPHY

Alexander JW: Surgical infections. Surg Clin North Am 60(1), February 1980
American College of Surgeons: Manual on Control of Infections in Surgical Patients. Philadelphia, Lippincott, 1976
Hunt TK: Wound Healing and Wound Infection. New York, Appleton-Century-Crofts, 1980

QUESTIONS

DIRECTIONS: Each of the questions or incomplete statements below is followed by five suggested answers or completions. Select the *one* that is *best* in each case.

A 40-year-old female who had a cholecystectomy three days ago suddenly develops severe chills, temperature of 104°F, hypotension, prostration, and leukocytosis. Blood culture grows *Serratia marcescens*.

1. The most likely cause of this complication is:
   A. Ascending cholangitis
   B. Subphrenic abscess
   C. Pulmonary atelectasis
   D. A contaminated intravenous catheter
   E. Bile peritonitis
2. The most appropriate antibiotic to be given after the above culture result is obtained is:
   A. Penicillin
   B. Ampicillin
   C. Gentamycin
   D. Clindamycin
   E. Cephalosporin
3. Complications of which to be aware when using this agent include:
   A. Hepatic necrosis
   B. Coombs'-positive hemolytic anemia
   C. Coombs'-negative hemolytic anemia
   D. Aplastic anemia
   E. Ototoxicity
4. Nosocomial infection usually involves the:
   A. Incision
   b. Respiratory tract
   C. Urinary tract
   D. Intravenous sites
   E. Deep veins of the leg

5. The offending bacterium in most contaminated respirators is:
   A. *Proteus*
   B. *Pseudomonas*
   C. *Staphylococcus*
   D. *Serratia*
   E. *Bacteroides*

DIRECTIONS: The group of items below consists of five lettered headings, followed by a list of numbered words or phrases. For *each* numbered word or phrase, select the *one* lettered heading or lettered component that is most closely associated with it. Each lettered heading or lettered component may be selected once, more than once, or not at all.

   A Chloramphenicol
   B Methicillin
   C Erythromycin
   D Tetracycline
   E Penicillin

---

6. Hepatic necrosis
7. Diarrhea, nausea, vomiting
8. *Salmonella*
9. Stains teeth in children
10. *Staphylococcus aureus*

DIRECTIONS: For each of the questions or incomplete statements below, *one* or *more* of the answers or completions given is correct. Select:

   A if only *1, 2, and 3* are correct
   B if only *1 and 3* are correct
   C if only *2 and 4* are correct
   D if only 4 is correct
   E if all are correct

---

11. Sensitivity results are irrelevant in the treatment of infections caused by:
    1. *Staphylococcus aureus*
    2. *Proteus mirabilis*
    3. *Escherichia coli*
    4. *Diplococcus pneumoniae*
12. *Bacteroides fragilis:*
    1. May cause septic thrombophlebitis
    2. Clindamycin is the antibiotic of choice
    3. Obligate anaerobe
    4. Rarely exists in mixed infections
13. Tends to decrease the incidence of postoperative wound infections:
    1. Depilatory preparation
    2. Prophylactic antibiotics begun immediately postoperatively and continued for at least one week

     3. Delayed primary skin closure
     4. Multistrand suture material
14. Problems associated with antibiotics include:
     1. Fungal superinfection
     2. Aplastic anemia
     3. Fever that resolves on discontinuation of therapy
     4. Pseudomembranous enterocolitis
15. Transient bacteremia has been demonstrated during minor procedures including:
     1. Bladder catheterization
     2. Sigmoidoscopy with biopsy
     3. Percutaneous liver biopsy
     4. Barium enema examination

ANSWERS

  1 **D** "Third day surgical fever" is iatrogenic bacteremia secondary to acute thrombophlebitis at an intravenous site. The organisms involved include *Serratia* (30 percent), *Klebsiella* (16 percent), *Bacteroides* (13 percent) and *Staphylococcus* (11 percent). Treatment includes removal of catheter and appropriate antibiotic therapy.

  2. **C** Gentamycin is appropriate for most Gram-negative bacteria.

  3. **E** Nephrotoxicity and ototoxicity are complications resulting from the use of genta, kana, neo, and strep.

  4. **C** Hospital-acquired infections have a prevalence of about 5 to 10 percent. Half of these involve the urinary tract, one-quarter involve the surgical wound, and one-fifth involve the lower respiratory tract. Most are Gram-negative infections

  5. **B** *Pseudomonas,* so-called water bacteria, thrive in distilled water used in inhalation therapy equipment.

  6. **D**

  7. **C**

  8. **A**

  9. **D**

10. **B**

11. **D** *D. pneumoniae* is always sensitive to penicillin.

12. **A.** *Bacteroides* may cause "third day surgical fever"; responds to clinda or chloro; cultures only under anaerobic conditions (not in routine media); is found often in mixed infections. It is a normal inhabitant of the lower intestinal tract, upper respiratory tract, and GU system.

13. **B** Depilatory preparation is superior to shaving; prophylactic antibiotics must be started preoperatively to be effective; monofilament suture does not have interstices, which harbor bacteria.

14. **E** All are correct.

15. **E** All are correct, but usually of no clinical significance.

28. Fluid, Electrolytes, and Nutrition

FLUID AND ELECTROLYTES

THREE OBJECTIVES OF FLUID THERAPY
1. Maintenance requirements
2. Replacement of ongoing losses
3. Replacement of previous losses

Normal Daily Maintenance Requirements
1. Water — 2500 ml (35 ml/kg)
2. Sodium — 100 mEq
3. Potassium — 60 mEq
4. Chloride — 100 mEq
5. Calories — 2000 (25–40 cal/kg)–fully achieved only with total parenteral nutrition (See page 294)

If this Patient then Requires Insertion of a Nasogastric (NG) Tube, his Intravenous Management Changes
1. Ongoing loss thru NG tube must be replaced
2. Replacement most accurately determined by measurement of electrolyte content of lost fluid
3. But determined in practice by estimation of these electrolytes from standard table based on actual fluid volume of loss (See Table 1)

If Patient Was Not Completely Healthy on Admission to the Hospital, but Had Sustained Unmeasured Fluid Losses (such as Vomiting or Diarrhea), Estimate what these Losses Were
1. Fluid deficit (liters)
   a. Mild dehydration = loss of 4 percent body weight (kg)
   b. Moderate = 6 percent
   c. Severe = 8 percent
2. Sodium (mEq): $(140 \times FD) + (140 - Na)$ (60 percent BW − FD) Where Na = serum sodium in mEq/L; FD = fluid deficit in L; BW = body weight in Kg

Table 1.   Content of Gastrointestinal Fluids (Approximate)

| | Volume | Electrolyte | | (mEq/l) | |
	l/day	Na	K	CL	HCO$_3$
Stomach	1.5	70	10	60	0
Bile	1	140	5	90	40
Pancreas	1	140	5	60	100
Small bowel	3	90	5	90	30
Diarrhea	—	120	25	90	45

In theory, once previous losses, ongoing losses and maintenance requirements have been estimated, it is possible to arrive at a volume of fluid, and millequivalants of sodium, potassium, chloride and bicarbonate. As a patient cannot simply drink a glass of water and take a teaspoon of each of these electrolytes, it is necessary to choose a bottle from the shelf which most closely meets these requirements
1. Solutions generally available
   a. Normal saline (NS) = 154 mEq Na/L; 154 mEq Cl/L
   b. 5 percent dextrose in water (D$_5$ W) = 200 calories/L
   c. Ringer's lactate (RL) = 130 mEq Na/L; 4 mEq K/L; 109 mEq Cl/L; 28 mEq HCO$_3$/L
   d. Several combinations of the above are also available (e.g., D$_5$ NS, D$_5$RL, D$_{10}$W, ½NS, D$_5$1/3NS, etc.)

After the amount and composition of fluid have been determined, determine the period of time over which it should be administered
1. By the urgency of the operation or clinical manifestation of deficits
   a. Within 2 hours: gangrenous bowel; septic shock
   b. Within 24 hours: perforated appendix, small bowel obstruction, cholecystitis
   c. Within several days: pyloric obstruction; common bile duct obstruction

The potential inaccuracy of this approach should be apparent. Guard against the inaccuracy of these calculations doing harm to the patient
1. Monitor the patient—adequate tissue perfusion is reflected by
   a. Good urine output
   b. Good mental status
   c. Rise of blood pressure to normal
   d. Fall of pulse to normal
   e. Normal CVP or PWP
   f. Normal serum electrolytes

If despite this treatment the patient develops an electrolyte abnormality, early recognition and prompt treatment are essential (See Table 2)

Table 2. Electrolytes and Acid-Base Disturbances

Abnormality	Usual Etiology	Clinical Findings	Treatment
Hypokalemia	*NG losses* Overhydration Diuretics Alkalosis	Muscle contractility decreases EKG: ↓ T, present U	KCL

Hyperkalemia	*Renal insufficiency*
	Catabolic states
	Addison's disease
		Minimal
		Abdominal pain,
		  nausea &
		  vomiting,
		↑ T, wide QRS, ST
		Cardiac arrest
			Dextrose and insulin
			Na HCO$_3$
			Ca gluconate
			Kayexelate
			Dialysis

Hyponatremia	*Overhydration*
	Inappropriate ADH
	Cirrhosis
	Salt-losing nephritis
		Mental obtundation
		Seizures
			Fluid restriction
			In cirrhosis,
			  treatment *not*
			  needed

Hypernatremia	*Dehydration*	Muscle tremors Seizures CNS ↓	Stop Na-containing fluids and drugs Give fluid (liters)- 60% BW × (140-Na) ——————— 140
Hypocalcemia	*Hypopara-* *thyroidism* Pancreatitis Renal insufficiency Tissue necrosis	↑ DTR's Abdominal cramps Prolonged Q-T Carpopedal spasm	Calcium gluconate Treat alkalosis

Hypercalcemia	*Cancer* with bony
	  metastases
	Primary hyper-
	  para-
	  thyroid etc.
		N/V/constipation
		Fatigue
		CNS ↓
			Saline
			Lasix
			Mithramycin
			Steroids
			Dialysis

Metabolic Acidosis	Ketoacidosis
	Lactic acidosis
	Renal tubular
	  acidosis
	Diarrhea
		Hyperventilation
		  (compensatory)
		CNS ↓
			Correct cause
			NaHCO$_3$ required
			  (mEq):
			30% BW × (25 −
			HCO$_5$)

Metabolic Alkalosis	NG losses
	Diuretic therapy
	Hyperaldos-
	  teronism
		Minimal
		compensatory
		hypoventilation
		Tetany
		CNS ↓
			Correct cause
			KCl to çorrect for
			  renal losses
			Ca for tetany

Most common electrolyte abnormality seen in patients on the surgical ward:

1. Hypokalemic hyponatremic, metabolic alkalosis due to NG suction or vomiting
2. Paradoxical aciduria (allows potassium retention, but in exchange for hydrogen excretion)
3. Rx: normal saline and potassium

SURGICAL NUTRITION

TOTAL PARENTERAL NUTRITION (INTRAVENOUS HYPERALIMENTATION)

Indications
1. Gastrointestinal failure
   a. Enterocutaneous fistula
   b. Prolonged ileus
   c. Chronic intestinal obstruction
2. Supplement to oral feedings in
   a. Severe burns
   b. Prolonged infection
3. Treatment of protein-calorie malnutrition prior to elective surgery
4. Treatment of uremia (essential amino acids)

d. Severe inflammatory
   bowel disease
e. Acute ulcerative colitis

Requirements in Adults
1. 25 to 40 cal/kg daily—increased with sepsis, peritonitis, burns, fractures
2. Carbohydrate—50 percent
3. Fat—30 to 40 percent
4. Protein—10 to 15 percent

Content
1. Approximately 1 calorie per cc
2. Gradually work up to 3 liters daily (3000 cal)
3. Commercial solutions include protein hydrolysate and 50 percent dextrose
4. Electrolytes include sodium chloride, sodium bicarbonate, potassium chloride, calcium chloride, potassium phosphate (especially in casein hydrolystate), magnesium sulfate
5. Fat-soluble vitamins (watch out for excess)—A, D, E, K
6. Water-soluble vitamins—B, C
7. Iron
8. Insulin

Complications
1. Catheter-related
   a. Technical problems during insertion (pneumothorax, etc.)
   b. Sepsis
      i. Usually *Staphylococcus epidermidis*
      ii. Candida in patients with multisystem disease
      iii. Treatment: removal of catheter
      iv. Prevention: local care, careful preparation of solutions, "TPN team," nonthrombogenic catheter materials, include small amount of heparin in solutions (one-half unit/cc)
2. Metabolic
   a. Hyperglycemia—treat with sliding scale insulin; watch for potassium deficit

b. Hypomagnesemia—neurologic symptoms, anorexia, nausea, vomiting
c. Azotemia—expecially in patients with renal or hepatic failure. Treat by using *essential* amino acids
d. Hyperosmolar nonketotic coma—due to dehydration caused by glycosuria, which results from inadequate insulin and total body potassium deficit
e. Hypoglycemia—if hyperalimentation stopped suddenly
f. Hyperchloremic metabolic acidosis—due to too much chloride and monohydrochloride in amino acid solutions
g. Hyperammonemia—especially in primary hepatic disorders; excessive ammonia in protein hydrolysate; arginine, ornithine, aspartine, or glutamate deficiency
h. Hypophosphatemia
   i. Etiology: intracellular accretion of phosphate from serum
   ii. Result
      1) Decline in red cell ATP and 2,3-DPG
      2) Impaired capacity of blood to deliver oxygen to tissues
      3) Muscular weakness, seizures, coma
   iii. Therapy: potassium dihydrogen phosphate 20 mEq per 1000 calories
i. Essential fatty acid deficiency
   i. Findings
      1) Desquamative dermatitis
      2) Hair loss
      3) Thrombocytopenia
      4) Poor wound healing
      5) Abnormal plasma lipid pattern
   ii. Cause: :two to four weeks of hyperalimentation without administration of fats
   iii. Treatment: Intralipid (10 percent solution)

"ARTIFICIAL GUT" (indwelling line for home use)

Indications
1. Short bowel syndrome
2. Severe Crohn's disease

Access
1. Silastic tube through subcutaneous tunnel to central vein (Hickman catheter)

Method
1. Self-administration at home using pump for continuous or overnight infusion of TPN

ELEMENTAL DIET

Indications
1. Substitute for TPN where part of gastrointestinal tract is still functional

Method: continuous drip via
1. Small nasogastric tube
2. Gastrostomy, or
3. Jejunostomy

Complications
1. Diarrhea—most with jejunostomy
2. Hypertonic dehydration
3. Dumping syndrome
4. Aspiration—especially with intragastric feedings if gag reflex absent

SELECTED BIBLIOGRAPHY

Carroll HJ, Oh MS: Water Electrolyte and Acid-base Metabolism. Philadelphia, Lippincott, 1978
Fischer JE (ed): Nutritional support in the seriously ill patient. Curr Probl Surg 17(1): September 1980
Mullen JL, et al.: Surgical nutrition. Surg Clin North Am 61(3): June 1981

QUESTIONS

A 30-year-old male develops a wound infection two days after a bowel resection for stab wound of the abdomen. Opening the skin results in a large amount of continuing drainage of small bowel content.
1. Initial therapy should include:
   A. Intravenous hyperalimentation
   B. Elemental diet
   C. Lactated Ringer's with dextrose
   D. Exploratory laparotomy and resection
   E. None of these
2. Barium study reveals a fistula of the distal ileum with no distal obstruction. Therapy at this point should include:
   A. Intravenous hyperalimentation
   B. Elemental diet
   C. Lactated Ringer's with dextrose
   D. Exploratory laparotomy and resection
   E. None of these
3. On the tenth postoperative day, this patient complains of weakness and paresthesias of his extremities. Twenty-four hours later, he sustains a seizure and falls into a coma. Blood gases are normal. Serum chemistries include sodium = 135 mEq/liter, potassium = 4.9 mEq/liter, chloride = 101 mEq/liter, creatinine = 1.2 mg percent, phosphate = 0.5 mg percent, calcium = 5.8 mg percent, blood urea nitrogen = 20 mg percent, magnesium = 1.4 mEq/liter. Appropriate therapy should include administration of:
   A. Sodium bicarbonate
   B. Diazepam (Valium)
   C. Inorganic phosphate

D. Hypertonic sodium chloride

E. Hemodialysis

4. The therapy indicated above may lead to a fall in serum:

A. Sodium

B. Potassium

C. Magnesium

D. Phosphate

E. Calcium

5. Prevention of hyperammonemia during TPN may include administration of:

A. Inorganic phosphate

B. Calcium

C. Arginine glutamate

D. Magnesium

E. Fructose

6. A 40-year-old female with known peptic ulcer disease is admitted with a five-day history of vomiting everything she eats. Physical examination reveals marked dehydration. Arterial blood gases are as follows: pH=7.62, pCO_2=54, pO_2=75. Which of the following substances is initially indicated to help correct this acid-base problem?

A. Calcium

B. Magnesium

C. Hydrogen

D. Bicarbonate

E. Potassium

7. A 30-year-old female requires total parenteral nutrition for Crohn's disease. During insertion of a subclavian catheter, the patient becomes dyspneic, with a respiratory rate of 32 per minute, pulse rate of 120 per minute, and a blood pressure drop to 80/60. Appropriate immediate action is:

A. Intubation and pressure-controlled respiration

B. Intubation and volume-controlled respiration

C. Tracheostomy

D. Chest x-ray and lung scan

E. Chest tube

8. A 50-year-old female with a history of congestive heart failure is admitted due to a perforated duodenal ulcer. She receives 500 cc dextrose in water over six hours and is then taken to the operating room. Upon induction of anesthesia her blood pressure drops to 80. The probable cause is:

A. Septic shock

B. Myocardial infarction

C. Inadequate depth of anesthesia

D. Hemorrhage

E. Hypovolemia

9. A 70-year-old male develops pancreatitis and acute tubular necrosis following splenectomy for trauma. He has chronic congestive heart failure. His fluid requirements are best determined by:

A. Daily weights

B. Accurate intake and output

C. Urine and serum osmolarity

  D. Wedge pressure monitoring
  E. Arterial pressure monitoring

ANSWERS

1. **A** Hyperalimentation is indicated in the treatment of small bowel fistulas to allow healing and prevent protein-calorie malnutrition.
2. **A** If a high small bowel or duodenal fistula were discovered, it might be possible to use an elemental diet through a jejunal tube; however, a low small bowel fistula requires continued intravenous hyperalimentation. Operative repair is reserved for those fistulas failing to heal on TPN, or those with distal obstruction.
3. **C** These symptoms are characteristic of hypophosphatemia. Treatment is by administration of potassium dihydrogen phosphate. This problem should not occur with casein hydrolysate, which contains phosphate, but fibrin hydrolysate may require supplementation with phosphate.
4. **E** Administration of phosphate will lead to a drop in calcium.
5. **C** Arginine increases the efficiency of the ammonia-urea cycle and is useful in preventing hyperammonemia.
6. **E** Gastric outlet obstruction and vomiting results in loss of water, sodium chloride, acid, and potassium. Renal conservation of potassium in exchange for hydrogen causes further acid loss (paradoxical aciduria). While hydration with saline is necessary, replacement of potassium is most important in reversing the metabolic alkalosis.
7. **E** The overall complication rate in the insertion of subclavian lines is 4 to 5%. The most frequent complication is pneumothorax induced by puncturing the pleura, which lies in close proximity to the subclavian vein. Physical examination alone should allow a rapid diagnosis and appropriate treatment, which is insertion of a chest tube on the involved side. It is not necessary to obtain a chest x-ray and intubation would just worsen the patient's symptoms. Avoidance of this problem requires attention to detail in the insertion of these lines. With the patient's head turned to the opposite side, the needle is inserted gradually through the skin and underneath the clavicle, aiming toward the suprasternal notch. If the line is not successfully inserted after a maximum of two or three attempts, the approach should be abandoned.
8. **E** A perforated ulcer leads to severe peritonitis and a large third-space loss of fluid. Volume replacement is the most significant preoperative procedure and requires large amount of fluid. If heart failure is a possibility, a Swan-Ganz catheter should be inserted to assess the state of hydration and monitor fluid replacement. In any case, 500 cc D_5W over six hours is inadequate.
9. **D** Pulmonary wedge pressure monitoring using a Swan-Ganz catheter is the method of choice for determining fluid requirements in this case because daily weights would not reflect third-space losses due to the pancreatitis, urine osmolarity is affected by the acute tubular necrosis, and arterial pressure changes occur only after major volume deficits.

29. Thermal Injuries

BURNS

FUNCTIONS OF INTACT SKIN

1. Prevents evaporative loss of water and electrolytes
2. Prevents bacterial invasion

CLASSIFICATION OF BURNS

1. *First degree:* erythema and edema, only epidermis involved
2. *Second degree:* blistering, part of dermis damaged, but sweat glands and part of dermis remain viable
3. *Third degree:* deep white color or charred black and leathery, complete destruction of dermis, sweat glands, sebaceous glands,and hair follicles. Cannot regenerate epithelium. Less painful because nerve endings destroyed

Note: Infection in second degree burn may cause loss of remaining dermis and convert it to third degree

ESTIMATION OF PERCENT OF BODY SURFACE BURNED

1. For adults, use "rule of nines" (See Fig. 29-1)
2. For infants, head is 19 percent of body surface and each lower extremity is 13 percent

COMPLICATIONS OF BURNS

Loss of Fluid and Electrolytes
1. Etiology
   a. Generalized increase in capillary permeability with loss into interstitial space (edema)
   b. Returns to normal in 48 hours with resorption of edema and diuresis
2. Treatment
   a. Monitor urine output and CVP
   b. Fluid therapy using standardized formula such as Brooke Army formula (calculate burns > 50 percent as 50 percent)

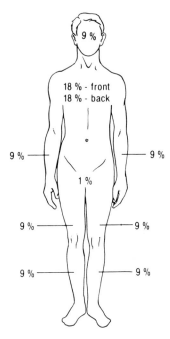

Figure 29-1 "Rule of Nines" to estimate percent of body surface burned.

    i. Colloid—0.5 cc per kg per percent burned for first 24 hours
    ii. Crystalloid Ringer's lactate—1.5 cc per kg per percent burned for first 24 hours
    iii. D_5W—2000 cc (adult)

Loss of Red Cells
1. Etiology
    a. Direct heat hemolysis
    b. Thrombosis of blood vessels with trapping of red blood cells
    c. Sequestration in reticuloendothelial system of damaged cells
    d. Sludging
2. Manifestations
    a. Initial increased hematocrit due to loss of plasma
    b. Later decreased hematocrit
    c. Free hemoglobin in urine
3. Therapy—transfuse when necessary, usually after 72 hours

Catabolism
1. Etiology
    a. Stimulation of adrenal cortical activity
    b. Nitrogen losses
2. Manifestation—weight loss approximately one pound per day
3. Therapy
    a. High protein, high calorie diet, or

    b. Nasogastric feedings, or
    c. Hyperalimentation

Decrease in Cardiac Output
1. Etiology
    a. Hypovolemia
    b. Circulating myocardial depressant factor
2. Therapy—fluid replacement

Paralytic Ileus
1. Manifestation—may lead to acute gastric dilatation with vomiting and aspiration
2. Therapy—nothing by mouth for two days

Curling's Ulcer
Therapy—antacids, cimetidine

Pulmonary Complications
1. Etiology
    a. Acute upper airway obstruction
    b. Inhalation injury—noxious products of combustion
    c. Postburn pulmonary insufficiency
    d. Atelectasis, pneumonia
    e. Respiratory compromise due to tight eschar (perform escharotomy)

Infection
1. Etiology
    a. Early—microorganisms from hair follicles and sweat glands (especially *Staphylococcus*)
    b. Later (fifth day)—gram-negative bacilli, especially *Pseudomonas aeruginosa*
    c. Impairment of inflammatory reaction—especially leukocyte chemotaxis and margination
    d. Later—opportunists (especially candida, aspergillus, phycomycetes); violaceous or black spots appear
2. Diagnosis
    a. Quantitative culture of burn tissue homogenate
    b. Histologic examination for fungi
3. Therapy—appropriate antibiotics
4. Prevention—adequate wound care by
    a. Exposure (especially face)
    b. Initial excision and grafting or tangential excision—however, the problem is determining accurately the depth of the injury
    c. Dressings—occlusive, absorptive, bulky, using
        i. Sulfamylon cream—10 percent
            1) Advantages—penetrates eschar wall, decreases evaporative water loss
            2) Disadvantages—pain on application, allergic reactions, carbonic anhydrase inhibitor, implies metabolic acidosis and tachypnea

    ii. Silver sulfadiazine
      1) Advantages—less pain, not carbonic anhydrase inhibitor
      2) Disadvantages—precipitation of sulfa crystals in renal tubules (rare)
    iii. Silver nitrate soaks—0.5 percent
      1) Disadvantages—stains black when exposed to light, difficult application, depletes and dilutes sodium, chloride, potassium, calcium
5. Aim in treatment of third degree burn—remove eschar and apply skin graft, which may be
    a. Split thickness—may use mesh dermatome to expand graft
    b. Allograft or porcine xenograft—will persist 15 to 30 days

Other Problems
1. Tetanus—prophylaxis
2. Pain—narcotics intravenously
3. Tight eschar—escharotomy

FROSTBITE

1. Theories of pathogenesis
    a. Vascular injury—vasoconstriction, vasodilatation, edema, sludging, thrombosis, necrosis
    b. Direct cold injury
2. Classification
    a. First degree—mottled, blue, purple, red, edema within three hours lasting to ten days
    b. Second degree—hyperemia, edema, vesicles, edema disappears within five days, black eschars form, throbbing and aching, underlying skin is thin, soft, easily injured
    c. Third degree—full thickness, ulceration, edema, burning, aching, throbbing pains, eschar desquamates, ulcer epithelializes
    d. Fourth degree—destruction of entire part including bone, paresthesias, dry gangrene, demarcates at about one month
3. Therapy
    a. Anticoagulants (debated)
    b. Sympathectomy or vasodilators (debated) in early frostbite, but of value for late complications (such as chilblain or causalgia)
    c. Rewarming in 90° to 104° Farenheit waterbath
    d. Loose dry dressing over vesicles, daily cleansing
    e. Tetanus toxoid, penicillin
    f. Absolute bed rest and elevation
    g. No smoking

h. Physical therapy, whirlpool therapy when eschar desquamated
i. Bivalve necrotic eschar on extremities
j. Amputation only for wet gangrene or when eschar separates and line of demarcation is clear

ELECTRICAL BURN

1. Usually deeper than apparent
2. Behaves like a crush injury

SELECTED BIBLIOGRAPHY

Pruitt BA Jr: The burn patient: I. Initial care. Curr Probl Surg 16(4): April 1979
Pruitt BA Jr: The burn patient: II. Later care and complications of thermal injury. Curr Probl Surg 16(5): May 1979

QUESTIONS

In a house fire a 34-year-old female sustains third degree burns over her entire anterior chest and abdomen and circumferentially around both arms and forearms.
1. What percent of body surface is involved?
   A. 54 percent
   B. 45 percent
   C. 36 percent
   D. 27 percent
   E. 18 percent
2. Initial therapy on arrival in the emergency room should include all of the following *except?*
   A. Insertion of central venous line
   B. Administration of colloids
   C. Tracheostomy
   D. Tetanus toxoid
   E. Intravenous morphine sulfate
3. The total volume of fluid therapy for the first 24 hours using the Brooke Army formula is approximately?
   A. 2.5 liters
   B. 3.5 liters
   C. 4.5 liters
   D. 5.5 liters
   E. 6.5 liters

4. The patient complains of severe thirst after four hours of intravenous therapy. Appropriate measures at this time include:
   A. Initiate regular diet
   B. Oral fluids as tolerated
   C. Check urine output, central venous pressure, and adjust rate of fluid administration if necessary
   D. Reassure patient, sedate if thirst continues
   E. Infuse hypertonic saline

5. If systemic antibiotic therapy is to be started on the first post-burn day, the most logical choice would be:
   A. Penicillin
   B. Tetracycline
   C. Gentamycin
   D. Clindamycin
   E. A combination of the above

6. The most common cause of burn wound sepsis is:
   A. *Staphylococcus aureus*
   B. *Pseudomonas aeruginosa*
   C. *Bacterioides fragilis*
   D. *Candida albicans*
   E. *E. coli*

7. Three weeks later, the patient develops hemorrhagic spots in the wound and a distended abdomen. A burn wound biopsy showing pseudohyphae most likely indicates:
   A. *Pseudomonas*
   B. Sporotrichosis
   C. *Candida*
   D. *Staphylococcus*
   E. *Proteus*

8. Complications associated with topical sulfamylon cream include all of the following *except:*
   A. Acidosis
   B. Pain
   C. Tachypnea
   D. Hyponatremia
   E. Allergic reaction

9. Although considerable controversy exists concerning appropriate *early* therapy in frostbite, which of the following is *least* likely to be indicated?
   A. Sympathectomy
   B. Rapid rewarming
   C. Bed rest and elevation
   D. Anticoagulants
   E. Early amputation

ANSWERS

1. **C**

2. **C** Insertion of an endotracheal tube or tracheostomy may be indicated in upper airway burns.

3. **E** By the Brooke Army formula, the total amount of fluid necessary for the first 24 hours is 0.5 cc × 60 kg × 36% burn = 1080 cc colloid, 1.5 cc × 60 kg × 36% burn = 3240 cc Ringer's Lactate, plus 2000 cc D_5W. This amounts to a total of 6320 cc in the first 24 hours.

4. **C** The patient indicating thirst is a sign that must be investigated to prevent further hypovolemia. Early paralytic ileus prevents oral intake for the first one or two days.

5. **A** Penicillin or a semisynthetic penicillin is indicated to prevent the most common cause of *early* burn wound sepsis, which is *Staphylococcus*. By the fifth day, the gram-negative bacilli predominate and the antibiotic may be switched at that time to gentamycin.

6. **B** The most common cause of sepsis originating from the burn wound is *Pseudomonas*. This is proven by quantitative culture of biopsied burn tissue.

7. **C**

8. **D** Hyponatremia is a common problem with silver nitrate soaks, not sulfamylon cream.

9. **E** The extent of tissue damage with frostbite may be deceiving on clinical examination during the early post-injury days. Often, later in the hospital course of such a patient, sloughing necrotic tissue will reveal viable tissue beneath it. Hence, early amputation is not usually performed.

30. Shock and Trauma

SHOCK

COMMON *MISCONCEPTIONS*

1. Shock is a single disease entity
2. In all stages and all types of shock, the physiologic defect is hypotension with low cardiac output and high peripheral resistance

DEFINITION

1. Basically, the result of inadequate tissue perfusion
2. Results from failure of the pump (heart), peripheral resistance, or perfusate (blood volume)

BASIC MECHANISM (at the capillary level)

1. Constriction of precapillary sphincters → arteriovenous shunting → reduced capillary blood flow → supranormal oxygen extraction → greater A-V O_2 difference → lower postcapillary venule pH
2. Hence, cellular anoxia occurs → release of vasoactive substances → dilatation of capillary channels → blood volume inadequate to fill large vascular bed → *stagnation, lactic acidosis, thrombosis* → cell death (at this point shock may be *irreversible*)
3. Bloodborne humoral depressant factor (debated)
   a. Transported via lymphatic channels into systemic circulation
   b. Does not easily cross blood-brain barrier
   c. Predisposes to destabilization of cell membranes
4. Order in which organ systems are deprived of blood flow:
   a. Skin and subcutaneous tissue first
   b. Intestine and skeletal muscle
   c. Major viscera (liver function usually good until terminal)
   d. Coronary and cerebral flow last
5. Compensatory mechanisms
   a. Hypovolemia → catecholamine release → vasoconstriction
   b. ↑ ADH and aldosterone → renal sodium and water retention
   c. Shift of interstitial fluid into vascular bed, sodium and water enter cells,

306

potassium leaves cells, enters into interstitial fluid. These are due to alteration of membrane transport (evidenced by low transmembrane potential difference) and result in cellular swelling
d. Hyperpnea, tachycardia

CLINICAL FINDINGS

1. Skin and mucous membranes—pale, cold, clammy with vasoconstriction; warm and dry with vasodilation
2. Muscle—weakness
3. Intestine—ileus
4. Renal—oliguria, anuria, high-output failure
5. Cerebral—depressed consciousness
6. Cardiac—increased output (especially in hyperdynamic septic shock)

Degree of shock	Blood pressure	Pulse	Thirst	Mental state	Skin
Mild	↓ 20%	Normal	Normal	Distressed	Cool, pale, slow response to pressure blanching (capillary filling)
Moderate	↓ 20–40%	Weak	Present	Apathetic	Cool, pale, slow response to pressure blanching
Severe	↓ over 40%	Very weak	Severe	Nearly comatose	Cold, ashen mottling, very sluggish response to pressure blanching

ETIOLOGIES

1. Hypovolemic—due to hemorrhage, third-space loss, burns. Results in ↓ CVP, ↑ peripheral resistance, tachycardia
2. Cardiogenic—due to cardiac arrhythmia, myocardial infarction, congestive heart failure. Results in ↑ CVP, ↑ peripheral resistance

3. Neurogenic—due to spinal anesthesia, quadriplegia. Results in sudden ↓ peripheral resistance, with pooling of blood in dilated capacitance vessels, ↑ heart rate
4. Septic—due to infection (usually gram-negative). Results in pooling of blood in microcirculation, ↑ capillary permeability, hypovolemia, ↓ peripheral resistance (A-V shunting). Also direct cardiotoxic effect. With gram-positive organism loss of fluid confined to infected area
5. Other causes—pulmonary embolism, inadequate cardiopulmonary bypass, anaphylaxis, insulin shock

MECHANISM OF SEPTIC SHOCK

Common Organisms Involved

Gram-positive	Gram-negative
D. pneumoniae	E. Coli
S. aureus	Enterobacter
Streptococci	Klebsiella
	Pseudomonas
	Proteus

Endotoxin (gram-negatives)
1. Direct endothelial damage due to activation of complement system initiating histamine and lysosome enzyme release
2. Interacts with neutrophils to liberate inflammatory substances and depletes neutrophil supply
3. Pyrogenicity (related to pyrogen production? hypothalamic effects?)
4. Bioassay for endotoxin—by Limulus polyphemus amebocyte gelation

TREATMENT OF SHOCK

Routine—goal is restoration of normal perfusion
1. Trendelenburg position
2. Ensure adequate airway
3. Monitor vital signs, urine output, NG suction
4. Control bleeding, splint fractures, etc.
5. Volume replacement if hypovolemic
   a. Best indication of adequacy of volume is pulmonary wedge pressure by Swan-Ganz catheter (measures left atrial pressure)
6. Transfuse if needed
   a. Major problem with massive transfusion is cold blood causing arrhythmias
   b. Watch for thrombocytopenia (dilutional)
   c. Watch for hypocalcemia (extracellular calcium deficit)
   d. While waiting for blood use plasma, saline, Ringer's lactate, Dextran

7. In long-term management, meet nutritional needs with hyperalimentation (2000 to 3000 cal daily)
8. Urea, diuretics, salt restriction for cerebral edema

Drugs
1. For acidosis—bicarbonate, tromethamine (THAM) (HCO_3^- distributed in a space about equal to twice extracellular fluid volume, i.e., 40 percent body weight)
2. For high peripheral resistance after volume replaced—vasodilators (phentolamine, phenoxybenzamine)
3. To correct intracellular energy substrate depletion
   a. Glucose, insulin, potassium (insulin potentiates transmembrane glucose transport
   b. Glucagon (activates adenylcyclase system to form cyclic AMP from ATP, effect potentiated by caloric loading)
   c. ATP infusion—improves myocardial function if membrane transport and intracellular processes are not irrevocably damaged
4. Cardiogenic shock—isoproterenol, dopamine, digitalis
5. Septic shock—antibiotics, hypothermic blanket, possible steroids to stabilize lysosomal membranes, replace inadequate adrenal function, etc.
6. Severe cardiogenic shock—intraaortic balloon pump

COMPLICATIONS

1. Postresuscitation hypertension: due to hypervolemia secondary to volume load, rapid mobilization of sequestered third space. Leads to respiratory failure, hematuria, encephalopathy
2. Pulmonary insufficiency (ARDS)
   a. Manifestations
      i. Hypoxemia unresponsive to inspired oxygen
      ii. Low compliance (stiff lung)
      iii. Diffuse interstitial edema pattern on chest x-ray
      iv. Fall in functional residual capacity
      v. Increase in cardiac output
      vi. Hyperventilation
      vii. Frequently associated with nonthoracic trauma
   b. Therapy
      i. Ventilatory support, careful monitoring
      ii. Positive end expiratory pressure (PEEP). Complication is fall in cardiac output, pneumothorax
3. Alterations in oxygen transport
   a. Background: (See Fig. 30-1) As oxygen tension rises, hemoglobin oxygen saturation rises in a sigmoidal-shaped curve. The P_{50} value is that tension at which saturation is 50 percent. This is normally about 27 mm Hg. Factors that shift the curve to the *right* (increase P_{50}) are *advantageous* in that an equivalent amount of oxygen can be *released* at a higher pO_2. Think about it

▶   i. Factors that increase P_{50} are increased: ("HAD A CAT")
        1) *H*emoglobin concentration
        2) *A*cid (i.e., decreased pH)
        3) *D*PG (results from thyroid hormone, increased pH, pyruvate kinase
            deficiency, increased inorganic phosphate, cortisol, young cell age)
        4) *A*TP
        5) *C*O$_2$
        6) *A*ldosterone
        7) *T*emperature (fever)
    ii. Factors that decrease P_{50}
        1) Opposite of above
        2) Carboxyhemoglobin
        3) Methemoglobin
    iii. Therapeutic implications—avoid:
        1) Too much old blood (decreased DPG concentration)
        2) Respiratory alkalosis (hyperventilation)
        3) Metabolic alkalosis (excess sodium bicarbonate)

TRAUMA

NECK TRAUMA

Clinical Findings
Note: even serious neck injuries may be ASYMPTOMATIC
1. Airway (larynx or trachea)
    a. Stridor

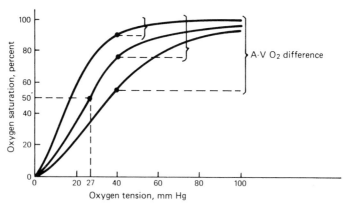

Figure 30-1 Oxygen–hemoglobin dissociation curves in normal (middle), rightward-, and leftward-shifted states. Normal P_{50} illustrated. Note that if arterial and venous oxygen tensions remain constant, arteriovenous oxygen difference increases if the curve shifts rightward.

    b. Hoarseness

    c. Dyspnea—airway compression by hematoma or aspiration of blood

    d. Subcutaneous emphysema

2. Esophagus

    a. Chest pain

    b. Dysphagia

    c. Usually associated with other injuries (e.g., spinal cord)

    d. Eventual sepsis from mediastinitis

3. Cervical spine or cord

    a. Paralysis

    b. Cervical pain or tenderness

    c. Diminished consciousness

4. Vascular injury

    a. External hemorrhage

    b. Hematoma

    c. Bruit (suggests arteriovenous fistula)

    d. Neurologic deficit—occurs with carotid injury if associated with hypotension or hypoxia

    e. Air embolism—occurs with venous injury

    f. Suspect carotid intimal disruption in blunt trauma with:

        i. Upper triangle hematoma

        ii. Horner's syndrome

        iii. Transient ischemia attacks

        iv. Lucid interval

        v. Monoplegia or hemiplegia in alert patient

5. Nerve injury

    a. Hypoglossal—tongue points to injury

    b. Bilateral vagus—hoarseness and dysphagia

    c. Phrenic—elevated hemidiaphragm

    d. Spinal accessory—paralysis of sternomastoid and deltoid

    e. Brachial plexus—sensory or motor deficits of upper extremity

Diagnosis

1. Rule out associated injuries
2. Neurologic examination
3. Chext x-ray—for widening of mediastinum
4. Lateral neck x-ray—may show anterior displacement of pharynx by air
5. Endoscopy—for suspected injury of larynx, pharynx, or esophagus
6. Gastrograffin swallow—for suspected esophageal injury
7. Arteriography—rarely required

Therapy

1. In emergency room

    a. Ensure airway—intubation, cricothyrotomy or tracheostomy may be indicated immediately

    b. Digital control of hemorrhage; intravenous fluids

    c. Immobilize if cervical spine injury suspected

2. In operating room (whenever platysma is penetrated)
   a. Prepare for cervicothoracic incision if wound near base of neck
   b. Obtain proximal and distal vascular control prior to exploring any hematoma surrounding a major vessel
   c. Keep head down until venous bleeding controlled, to prevent air embolism

Operative Approach for Specific Injuries
   a. Trachea or larynx
      i. Immediate tracheostomy for airway obstruction
      ii. Otherwise, suture, place tube through wound as tracheostomy, or perform end-to-end anastamosis
      iii. Temporary silastic stent for thyroid cartilage injury
   b. Esophagus—suture and drainage; pass NG tube to locate problem
   c. Cervical spine or cord—immobilize; decompression laminectomy may be required
   d. Carotid artery
      i. Repair after debridement; may use autogenous vein
      ii. If neurologic deficit has already occurred, LIGATE, DO NOT REPAIR—revascularization may cause fatal hemorrhagic infarction
   e. Vertebral artery
      i. Ligate—repair is difficult
      ii. Ligation; however, results in 2–3 percent incidence of fatal midbrain or cerebellar infarction
   f. Venous injury
      i. Keep head down until bleeding controlled by ligation
      ii. If air embolism occurs:
         1) Place left side down—this keeps air out of right ventricular outflow tract
         2) Trendelenburg position–this increases pulmonary perfusion and prevents further air embolism
         3) Maintain circulation by cardiac massage if necessary
         4) Aspirate air after advancing CVP line into heart
         5) Stop nitrous oxide—enters air bubble rapidly
   g. Lymphatic injury—ligate
   h. Nerve injury—neurorraphy

CHEST TRAUMA

1. Rib fracture
   a. Minor—symptomatic—observation, strapping
   b. Flail chest = portion of chest wall isolated by multiple rib fractures that moves paradoxically with respiration—requires ventilator for two to three weeks
2. Hemo- or penumothorax: immediate chest tube to underwater drainage
   a. Sucking wounds—occlusive dressing

     b. Indications for thoracotomy:
       i. Rapid bleeding (over 100 to 200 ml hourly)
       ii. Continued bleeding (over 1 liter total)
     c. Intercostal vessel is usual source of bleeding
3. Ruptured bronchus: persistant air leak or pneumomediastinum—repair or resection
4. Aortic tear
     a. Usually just distal to left subclavian at ligamentum arteriosum
     b. Urgent aortography and operative repair (few make it to hospital alive)
5. Heart: pericardiocentesis for immediate relief of tamponade, then operative repair
6. Diaphragm (almost always on left side): operative repair; if unrecognized, may present years later with herniation
7. Pulmonary contusion
     a. Findings: blood-tinged secretions, dyspnea, cyanosis, lung "white-out" on x-ray
     b. Treatment: fluid restriction, Swan-Ganz catheter, respiratory care
8. Adult Respiratory Distress Syndrome (ARDS, "Shock lung"): presents within one week of injury or resulting from septic complications; treatment is fluid restriction and positive end expiratory pressure (PEEP) ventilation
9. Thoracoabdominal injury (especially penetrating wounds): mortality very high if unrecognized; abdominal paracentesis and lavage useful
10. Esophagus
     a. Findings: pain, fever, subcutaneous emphysema, mediastinal "crunch" (Hamman's sign)
     b. Confirmation: chest x-ray—mediastinal widening or pneumomediastinum, left pleural effusion; gastrograffin swallow—false negatives common
     c. Treatment: nasogastric tube
       i. Recognized early—closure and drainage
       ii. Recognized late (after 48 hours)—must buttress closure and drain well

ABDOMINAL TRAUMA

Diagnosis and Immediate Treatment
1. Airway, breathing, circulation
2. Detailed history and physical; frequent vital signs
3. Intravenous fluid resuscitation
4. Type and cross, hematocrit, urinalysis
5. Nasogastric tube, Foley catheter
6. Locate all exit and entry wounds
7. Immobilize fractures (*beware:* cervical spine fracture)
8. X-ray: chest and abdomen; localize bullet—may have embolized
9. IVP for hematuria; possible cystogram
10. For stable patient with suspected retroperitoneal injury—amylase,

gastrograffin series, sonography, x-ray lumbar spine, IVP, angiography
11. Chest tube if indicated
12. Antibiotics for penetrating or visceral damage

Indications for Paracentesis and Lavage
1. Paracentesis for equivocal abdominal signs (> 100,000 cells/ml = positive)
2. Lavage if paracentesis is negative

Indications for Laparotomy
1. Peritoneal signs
2. Active bleeding (exclude blood loss elsewhere, especially pelvic fracture)
3. All gunshot wounds (somewhat controversial)
4. Positive tap or lavage

Performance of Laparatomy for Trauma
1. Long midline incision
2. Control bleeding (spleen, liver, pelvic vessels, mesenteric vessels)
3. Search for other injuries; try to avoid spillage from injured bowel
4. Explore only expanding or large retroperitoneal hematomas if blunt trauma; all retroperitoneal hematomas if penetrating trauma (Reason: renal bleeding secondary to blunt trauma is best controlled by an intact retroperitoneum)
5. Reflect hepatic flexure of colon and duodenum to look for duodenal or pancreatic injury

Specific Organs
1. Kidney: conserve as much tissue as possible; preoperative IVP important in evaluating function of contralateral kidney; if associated injuries require more rapid procedure, nephrectomy may be necessary
2. Ureter: (from simplest to most complex procedure)
   a. Transverse suture
   b. Resection and end-to-end anastomosis
   c. Ureteroneocystostomy
   d. Ureteroureterostomy
   e. Autotransplantation of kidney to pelvis
3. Bladder: suture; suprapubic cystostomy; drain perivesical space
4. Urethra: indwelling catheter alone if possible; otherwise, explore bladder
5. Spleen: attempt splenorraphy; otherwise, splenectomy
6. Gallbladder: cholecystectomy
7. Common bile duct (possible procedures)
   a. T-tube
   b. Anastomosis over T-tube
   c. Roux-en-Y choledochojejunostomy
8. Pancreas (DRAIN ALL)
   a. Tail—distal pancreatectomy
   b. Contusion—drain
   c. Head—pancreatectomy or pancreaticoduodenectomy
9. Stomach: debride and suture

10. Duodenum: duodenostomy with transverse closure, resection and anastomosis; for ampullary lesion, Whipple may be required
11. Small bowel: transverse suture, or resection and anastomosis
12. Colon:
    a. Clean—close primarily
    b. More extensive—resection with diverting colostomy; colostomy and mucous fistula; Hartmann's procedure; exteriorization
13. Rectum: Debridement and irrigation, perineal drainage, diverting colostomy

SELECTED BIBLIOGRAPHY

Oakes DD: Splenic trauma. Curr Probl Surg 18(6): June 1981
Trunkey DD: Trauma. Surg Clin North Am 62(1): February 1982
Williams JW, Sherman RT: Penetrating wounds of the neck: Surgical management. J Trauma 13:435, 1973

QUESTIONS

1. A 24-year-old female without neurologic deficits undergoes neck exploration for a stab wound. Massive hemorrhage appears to be arising from avulsion of the thyrocervical trunk off the subclavian artery. After packing to achieve tamponade, appropriate management is
   A. Division and ligation of subclavian artery
   B. Disarticulation of clavicle at sternoclavicular joint
   C. Repair through neck incision
   D. Transection of clavicle in its midportion
   E. Splitting sternum into second or third interspace
2. After appropriate management of that injury, a hole is found in the internal jugular vein. As it is being explored a massive venous air embolism occurs. Appropriate immediate management is to place the patient
   A. Left side down and head tilted downward
   B. Left side down and head tilted upward
   C. Right side down and head tilted downward
   D. Right side down and head tilted upward
   E. In Trendelenburg position
3. A 22-year-old man is noted to have hematuria following an automobile accident. An IVP delineates the caliceal systems well, but the left kidney shadow is enlarged, suggesting a perirenal hematoma. The lower urinary tract is normal. Appropriate treatment at this time is
   A. Laparotomy and partial nephrectomy
   B. Laparotomy and evacuation of the hematoma
   C. Renal scan
   D. Observation
4. A 30-year-old male is admitted with a gunshot wound of the left chest in the midaxillary line. Blood pressure is 90/60, pulse 120, respirations 30 per minute. After 2 liters of normal saline intravenously, central venous

pressure rises to 30 cm water but hypotension continues. Chest is clear and breath sounds normal. The most likely diagnosis is

A. Ruptured pulmonary artery
B. Myocardial infarction
C. Cardiac tamponade
D. Flail chest
E. Tension pneumothorax

5. The driver of a car involved in a head-on collision is found to have multiple rib fractures with pneumothorax, hemothorax, and flail chest. After resuscitation with intravenous fluids his blood pressure and pulse are normal, but his blood gases taken with 40 percent oxygen by face mask are: $pO_2=60$ mm Hg, $pCO_2=50$ mm Hg, Ph=7.31. Proper management at this point is

A. Increase the oxygen to 50 percent
B. Increase the oxygen to 100 percent
C. Introduce an endotracheal tube and use 40 percent oxygen by T-piece
D. Introduce an endotracheal tube and attach patient to volume control respirator

6. A 35-year-old male sustains multiple rib fractures in an airplane crash. On admission he is confused, hypoxic, and dyspneic. Appropriate treatment is

A. Chest strapping
B. Internal fixation of fractured ribs
C. Pericardiocentesis
D. Intubation and use of a pressure-controlled ventilator
E. Intubation and use of a volume-controlled ventilator

7. A 40-year-old male is brought to the hospital after an automobile accident and found to have progressive mediastinal and subcutaneous emphysema. Even after insertion of a chest tube he continues to have respiratory distress and a large air leak from the tube. The next step in his management is

A. Contrast bronchography
B. Median sternotomy
C. Esophagogram
D. Arch aortogram
E. Bronchoscopy

A 26-year-old female is admitted with a temperature of 104°F. An infected fetus is aborted and she develops tachypnea in the intensive care unit, where she is found to have a WBC of 2,600/cu mm and warm, dry skin.

8. The most likely diagnosis is:
A. Transient bacteremia
B. Major hemolytic reaction
C. Shwartzman reaction
D. Pulmonary embolism
E. Septic shock

9. Each of the following treatments might be indicated *except:*
A. Whole blood
B. Ringer's lactate
C. Levarterenol (Levophed)

    D. Isoproterenol (Isuprel)
    E. Antibiotics
10. A 59-year-old male with a ruptured appendix and history of congestive heart failure develops bibasilar rales and oliguria several hours postoperatively. His central venous pressure is normal. Which of the following studies would be most helpful in further management of this patient?
    A. Serum osmolarity
    B. Urine/serum creatinine ratio
    C. Arterial blood gases
    D. Electrocardiogram
    E. Pulmonary wedge pressure
11. Rapid, massive whole blood transfusion is most likely to produce immediate problems by virtue of its
    A. Low temperature
    B. Lack of calcium
    C. Citrate anticoagulant
    D. High potassium level
    E. Acidosis
12. The most likely cause of pneumothorax in a patient with adult respiratory distress syndrome is
    A. Arteriovenous shunting
    B. Volume-controlled ventilation
    C. Pressure-controlled ventilation
    D. Prolonged use of 100 percent oxygen
    E. Positive end expiratory pressure ventilation
13. The one defect common to all forms of shock is
    A. Hypotension
    B. Falling right atrial pressure
    C. Inadequate tissue perfusion
    D. Reduction in cardiac output
    E. Fall in left atrial pressure

ANSWERS

1. **E** Subclavian artery injuries are best approached through a combined cervicothoracic incision to allow safe repair.

2. **A** Venous air embolism is treated by placing the patient left side down and head tilted downward to discourage air from entering the right ventricular outflow tract. Obviously, the source of air must be immediately closed and resuscitation initiated.

3. **D** A small perirenal hematoma is probably well tamponaded by an intact retroperitonium and, in the absence of other injuries, requires observation only.

4. **C** A falling blood pressure and rising central venous pressure is indicative of cardiac tamponade. Distended neck veins and pulsus paradoxicus are confirmatory signs. Appropriate treatment is needle pericardiocentesis.

5. **D** Inadequate oxygenation in a patient with multiple chest injuries is treated best with endotracheal intubation and use of a ventilator. Tracheostomy is necessary only in the face of injuries obstructing the airway or after prolonged endotracheal intubation.

6. **E** Flail chest is best treated by mechanical ventilation using a volume-controlled system. It would be difficult for a patient with this injury to trigger a pressure-controlled ventilator.

7. **E** These are the typical manifestations of a rupture of a major bronchus or the trachea. Bronchoscopy will reveal the site of injury, which is usually in the lower thoracic trachea, bifurcation, or in the proximal major bronchi. After determination of the site of rupture, emergency thoracotomy is performed for repair of the laceration.

8. **E** Septic shock is characterized by decreased peripheral resistance, hypotension resulting in tachycardia, tachypnea causing a respiratory alkalosis, and fluid extravasation from the interstitial space into the intravascular compartment thereby increasing blood volume. Clinically, these mechanisms lead to a hypoperfused patient with warm extremities but oliguria and CNS depression. In later phases, vasoconstriction occurs, poor peripheral perfusion, lactic acidosis, then cell swelling and death.

9. **C** Although a vasopressor such as levarterenol would initially cause a rise in blood pressure, its critical effect is vasoconstriction, further depriving ischemic tissues of their blood supply. Isoproterenol, on the other hand, is a beta-stimulator that will increase cardiac output and not cause vasoconstriction.

10. **E** In determining fluid requirements in a patient with volume problems but cardiac disease, the best indication of state of hydration is the left atrial pressure, which can be measured by inserting a transvenous catheter through the right heart into the pulmonary artery, inflating its balloon, and measuring pulmonary artery wedge pressure (Swan-Ganz catheter). It is more accurate than right atrial pressure (CVP).

11. **A** The major immediate problems resulting from massive banked blood transfusion relate to low temperature causing cardiac arrhythmias.

12. **E** Positive end expiratory pressure (PEEP) is used to maintain alveoli open in the face of adult respiratory distress syndrome (shock lung syndrome) but may lead to pneumothorax or reduction in cardiac filling.

13. **C** Shock *is* inadequate tissue perfusion.

Index